The Internet for Radiology Practice

T0185052

Springer
New York
Berlin
Heidelberg
Hong Kong
London
Milan
Paris
Tokyo

THE
INTERNET
FOR
RADIOLOGY
PRACTICE

With 33 Illustrations

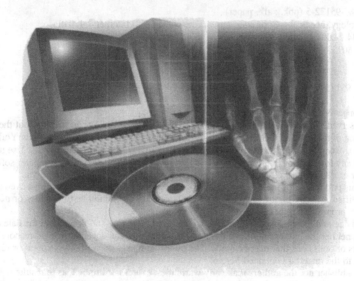

AMIT MEHTA, M.D.
Massachusetts General Hospital
Boston, Massachusetts
USA

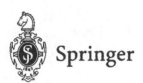
Springer

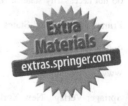
Extra
Materials
extras.springer.com

Amit Mehta, M.D.
Massachusetts General Hospital
Boston, MA 02114
USA
mehta@helix.mgh.harvard.edu

Library of Congress Cataloging-in-Publication Data

Mehta, Amit.
    The Internet for radiology practice / Amit Mehta.
        p. cm.
    Includes bibliographical references and index.

Additional material to this book can be downloaded from http://extras.springer.com.

    ISBN 0-387-95172-5 (pbk. : alk. paper)
        1. Radiology, Medical—Computer network resources.   2. Internet.   I. Title.
    R907 .M44   2003
    025.06′6160757—dc21

                                                                                2001031423

ISBN 0-387-95172-5   Printed on acid-free paper.

Printed in the United States of America.

9 8 7 6 5 4 3 2 1   SPIN 10788820

www.springer-ny.com

Springer-Verlag   New York Berlin Heidelberg
A member of BertelsmannSpringer Science+Business Media GmbH

To my family—Mom, Dad, Chetan, and Sonal—
for their unconditional support and love.

To my mentors—Keith, Dave, Murray, and Jim—
for their guidance.

To my friends—Nik, Neal, and Angela—
for their constant humor.

Series Preface

The Internet is the ultimate amalgamation of the Information Age and the Communication Age. It is a technology that took 40 years to become an overnight sensation, moving from the province of computer geeks to household utility in short order, once it was discovered. We have gone from thinking a URL was a form of alien presence to viewing it as a natural footnote to bus advertising.

Like the Internet itself, interest in computing, both local and distant, has grown exponentially. Now grandmothers send e-mails to their stockbrokers, meals are planned and the groceries purchased across the Web, and music videos can be previewed or concert tickets purchased—all with the help of the Internet. When our children come home from school, they are as likely to sign on to the Internet as they are to turn on the television. The Internet is a universal commodity, for those with access.

The American Internet User Survey found that more than 41.5 million adults in the United States actively are using the Internet. Of these Web users, 51% use the Web on a daily basis. It seems everybody needs to be connected to the Web, just as everybody seems to need to make cell-phone calls while changing lanes in heavy traffic. The Internet is nothing less than a library card to the world. At the most basic level, the Internet is a high-speed web of worldwide computer-based information resources connected together. It is a network of computer networks. One moment you can be browsing through the Library of Congress or looking at pictures from the National Library of Medicine, and the next moment conversing with a colleague in Indonesia.

What about the Internet and medicine? Well, we physicians sell information. That is what we do in medicine. That is what we always have done. Today, the difference is that we do it in an age built on information. Information, medical and otherwise, is all around us. From pocket pagers that deliver stock quotes and sports scores to palm-top digital assistance that wirelessly connects to the Internet, information is achieving the status of oxygen—it is all around us and invisible. (Oxygen also is the name of a computing project at the Massachusetts Institute of Technology that is aimed at achieving this goal.) Today, information is managed, moved, and organized in ways never thought of in the past and will soon be managed in ways not yet conceived. In medicine, information is vital, but the exponential growth of knowledge available requires new approaches to its dissemination, access, and use. Central to this is the Internet. Information is now the province of anyone with a computer. This has led to "disintermediation": the ability of consumers to go directly to the source of information (or goods and services), bypassing the intermediate steps of providers. In medicine, this means that physicians obtain and distribute information in new ways, patients obtain and receive their information in new ways, and, together, patients and providers interact in new ways. Very little has remained the same, and yet fundamentally nothing is different—we still sell information. Medicine has frequently led the way with new technology: we used print materials when books were in their infancy; we embraced the telephone like few other professions; pagers, two-way radio, and teleconferencing (telemedicine) were all adopted by medicine early in their development. The need for information always has driven this adoption, and it is no different for the Internet.

This series of texts on the Internet in medicine and in medical subspecialty areas is intended to assist in this natural evolution in two ways. First, it will help us understand the abilities of the Internet and know its tools so that we may capitalize on what the Internet holds for ourselves as physicians and our patients. Second, the medical applications of the Internet have grown too rapidly and are too specialty specific to explore in depth in any single volume. Hence, the birth of specialty-specific volumes. When the first edition of *The Internet for Physicians* was published, it was mainly the technophile fringe that was surfing the Web. The first edition attempted to introduce the concept of information transfer and communication and point the way toward a tool of the future. The second edition attempted to assuage trepidation in the use of this emerging tool and suggest the whys and wherefores of being connected. The needs that drove those goals almost have completely disappeared. The third edition is more focused on the medical aspects of the Internet and its use and much less on the nuts and bolts of connecting and communicating through the Web. This evolution has opened the possibility of a special series dedicated to the Internet in various specialties of medicine. Each of these specialty volumes deals with specialty-specific aspects of the Internet, going beyond the general scope of *The Internet for Physicians*. Each author has been chosen for his or her expertise in medical computing, and they are each a recognized leader in their field. Each volume builds on fundamentals introduced in *The Internet for Physicians*. While the volumes stand alone, they have all been created so that each fits within the same concept. As authors, we hope that this series will open new and exciting options for this new age of medical information. Surf's up!

Roger P. Smith, M.D.
University of Missouri–Kansas City School of Medicine
Kansas City, Missouri, USA
Author of *The Internet for Physicians*

Preface

A revolution has occurred. The world has and continues to become linked electronically from continent to continent and from coast to coast. The opportunity to communicate, exchange information, and promote new ideas has blossomed due to the development and distribution of the Internet. The Internet has allowed individuals from disparate geographic locations to share ideas, conduct transactions, and generate new paradigms for executing daily functions.

Radiology, a specialty that centers around data in the forms of both images and reports, is well suited to harness the power of the Internet. The features and benefits an electronic network provides to radiologists both personally on a day-to-day basis and as a collaborative specialty are endless. As the digital department becomes a reality, an intimate knowledge of the Internet and its affiliated technologies will become a necessity.

This book came about because of the overwhelming need to educate radiologists and personnel affiliated with the radiology practice about the Internet. The ability to utilize the offerings currently available and to develop applications for this technology promises to make radiologists, technologists, and administrators more effective in their professions. It allows radiologists to better help referring physicians and ultimately their own patients. It allows technologies to improve the efficiency of producing images. It allows administrators to make the practice more cost-effective and streamlined, allowing more patients to benefit from the offered services.

Initially, when the concept of this text was generated, the Internet revolution had just begun. Many people, including radiologists, were leaving their practices to join the "dot-com" revolution. Companies not only were finding new ways to do things using the Internet but also refining and restructuring many of the classic tasks for an electronic format. Over the course of writing the text, the Internet-affiliated technologies such as PACS, voice recognition, and Web-based distribution of images have become realities and fall under the rubric of Internet technologies; understanding these technologies is essential. Thus, the scope of the book grew to include what are deemed to be key and integral technologies for radiology practice in the coming decade.

My hope is that this book will familiarize the reader with the technology behind the Internet and provide a basic understanding of what radiologists need to know to gain the most out of its potential offerings. The text is in no way meant to serve as a comprehensive review of the entire Internet or its adjunct technologies, as individuals spend entire careers on these subjects; furthermore, there are comprehensive texts available on each of these subjects that will serve as an invaluable reference tool for the reader interested in further information. This text is meant to build a foundation and excite and encourage readers to go out and gain more understanding of the Internet and its adjunct technologies. I hope readers enjoy it and find it useful. As always, kudos or criticisms always are welcome.

Amit Mehta, M.D.
mehta@helix.mgh.harvard.edu

Contents

Part II: Tools of Utility

3. General Applications Every Radiologist Will Use

4. Electronic Education: Teaching Files and the Internet

Part III: Technologies Revolutionizing Radiology

5. PACS: Picture Archiving and Communication Systems

6. Teleradiology

7. Voice Recognition

8. Electronic Medical Record and Patient Care
Specific to Radiology

Part IV: Resources

9. Radiology Web Sites

Part V: Appendices

Appendix 1: ACR Standard for Digital Image Data Management

Appendix 2: ACR Standard for Teleradiology

Introduction

The planet is getting connected. At a pace unparalleled by any other technology in the history of the human race, the Internet has begun to connect people of various backgrounds, cultures, locations, and interests. It has provided a medium with which to communicate, share, learn, trade, and do business. The Internet is a technology that has the potential to impact each individual on the planet in a different way: for the educator, it can help gather information; for the business pundit, it can help trade stocks; for the physician, it can help treat patients.

The Internet specifically has had a great impact on the practice of radiology and on the radiologist. There are many aspects from which all physicians benefit, such as the use of Medline and other journal catalog functions to acquire up-to-date information on treating patients. Specific to radiology, however, the Internet has enabled the proliferation, installation, and acceptance of adjunct technologies, such as picture archiving and communication systems (PACS), the electronic medical record (EMR), teleradiology, and voice recognition (VR). Each of these technologies has begun to and promises to continue to improve both the efficiency with which we practice and the care we can provide to patients. The Internet allows us to collaborate with our colleagues in other countries for research, to consult with experts in difficult cases, and to teach students with our teaching files.

The number of radiology-specific Web sites just five years ago numbered in the thirties. A recent compilation numbers them in the thousands. Students, residents, and staff are all "wired," and this improves all facets of our specialty. Each day brings new uses for the Internet, both in academic and commercial applications. Companies and health care providers continue to offer information on-line in the form of Web pages, e-mail, and newsgroups. While many of the technologies we use in our practice on a daily basis have undergone scientific validation, clinical trials, and Food and Drug Administration (FDA) approval, the Internet is one of a small handful of technologies that have not begged for rigorous scientific validation prior to their widespread acceptance. A large part of the Internet's early and continued acceptance is due to its obvious utility and current ubiquity. The Internet, through its years of development, has grown and matured; its early uses are somewhat different from those of today. In addition, with the growth of the number of on-line users, the Internet community becomes stronger. Each day, new uses for the network concept and for the transfer of information in many forms to members on the network are being discovered.

As radiologists, we are at the forefront of experimenting with utilizing, and applying new technologies. It is required that we be able to combine this expertise with imaging and information technology (IT) and its applications. Within our specialty, computer technology and the Internet have revolutionized the way we work on a daily basis. The radiologic report, distributed to the referring physician previously on paper, can now be communicated in a myriad of electronic means at a pace deemed impossible by the previous methods. We are able to talk on the phone, e-mail over the Internet, videoconference over dedicated systems, and fax, to name a few alternatives. The radiologic examination, previously distributed on film, has become digital and can be transmitted anywhere using electronic connection lines. The many technologic advances we have seen in our lifetime have helped streamline our day-to-day practice and have enabled more concentrated effort on furthering many other aspects of radiology.

Interestingly, our patients are beginning to access the Internet as well. They are well informed about our methods and techniques. They challenge us to improve our skills and to innovate to create new ones. They are empowered and understand the consequences and options that they have at their disposal. They can now make educated additions to their care and can often help guide their physician to arrive at an optimum treatment plan. Much of the information is provided by our governing bodies (*www.radiologyresource.org*), while a portion of the information also comes from health care consumers themselves.

What follows is a brief summary of each chapter, which will guide you in your use of this book. We have seen the growth of the use of the computer in every facet of our lives. In the same way, we are beginning to see the utility and growth of the use of the Internet. But, beyond our personal lives, the enabling power of this technology for our professional lives is awesome. In Chapter 1, the background and history of the Internet, in addition to the concepts that govern its use and creation, are discussed. The ideas and technologies that make the Internet so useful are explained, and the building blocks that create the network are reviewed.

In Chapter 2, the necessary tools needed by the radiologist to get onto the Information Highway are discussed. If you already own a computer, this chapter will help you to refine your hardware elements. If you do not own a computer, this chapter will help you as a radiologist select the necessary components. This chapter also will explain the various options you have as a user to connect to the internet and will familiarize you with much of the language you will need in order to discuss these issues with vendors.

In Chapter 3, the various applications and software that are used in relation to the Internet are explored, including e-mail, browsers, and news groups. At the conclusion of this chapter, you will know what tools you should have on your computer in order to fully use the power of the Internet. With these tools you will be able to communicate, collaborate, and create with the help of your colleagues.

Many current users on the Internet explore the realm of on-line education and teaching files. In Chapter 4, the basic concepts behind creating a radiologic teaching file as well as using an on-line teaching file are discussed. Much of the use of the Internet in the past several years has been focused on the development of on-line education, usually in the form of teaching files.

The concepts of the Internet enable digital imaging and the creation of the digital department, a department in which no hard-copy film is produced. All image data are created in the forms of bits and bytes and shuttled on wires to monitors where we can view them. In Chapter 5, the technology and concepts of picture archiving and communication systems (PACS) are reviewed. PACS technology has revolutionized many facets of our practice. It has brought about new ways of viewing images, with three-dimensional (3D) stack formats to view two-dimensional (2D) images to frank 3D imaging. It has changed work-flow patterns, decreased the instances of lost film, and improved patient communication by providing complete availability around the clock. The PACS technology can make us more efficient as well as improve our ability to interpret image data, both of benefit to the patient.

Telemedicine and teleradiology are natural extensions of the digital department and are explored in Chatper 6. This technology has provided a new way for us to extend our reach as radiologists and improve patient care by allowing our expertise to geographically extend into global areas heretofore inaccessible to our subspecialty. We are now able to help underserviced areas as well as provide subspecialty care to centers that lack this luxury. Teleradiology will enable us to deal with the increasing demand for radiologic services into the next decade as the baby boomer population begins to enter a stage of health care consumption that will be the largest ever to tax the health care system.

Interestingly, the birth of these new technologies that are very much dependent on the Internet has spawned other adjunct technologies, such as three-dimensional imaging, data mining, resource utilization, practice management tools, as well as educational tools, including on-line textbooks, references, compendiums, and teaching files. All of these other technologies help to make the practice of radiology more efficient, exciting, and evolutionary.

In Chapter 7, voice recognition, a promising new spin-off technology that only could become a reality with the concepts of the Internet providing an infrastructure, is discussed. The integration of a system that transcribes and finalizes a report in real time serves to decrease the turnaround time of a final report to the referring physician and ultimately to the patient, thus improving the standard of care. It also reduces errors and improves overall efficiency while decreasing costs. The report can be made instantaneously available to a referring physician through an electronic medical record system (EMR). Voice recognition continues to improve as a technology and also soon will become ubiquitous. In the current climate of economic health care in which resources are scarce, solutions such as voice recognition (VR) help save funds and allow redirection of resources to other endeavors that ultimately benefit patient care.

With the advent of digital imaging and the progression of other fields of medicine into electronic-based records, from lab and report systems already in place to more image intensive systems, the electronic medical record is becoming a reality. In Chapter 8, the growing field of EMR is discussed. The development of this system, which can house all the necessary patient information from history and physical to pathology, radiology, and images from clinical medicine, promises to make the practice of medicine and radiology easier. An EMR solution ensures the integrity of data as well as allows instantaneous access to relevant data in any location at any time. This entire infrastructure is enabled by the Internet and network technologies. These are technologies that are a reality today in many medical centers and that are providing physicians with tangible improvements in patient care.

Chapter 9 provides an expansive and inclusive listing of radiology Web sites. Included are portal sites, sites offering teaching files and continuing medical education (CME) credit, modality sites, journal and publication sites, magazine sites, division and department sites, equipment vendor sites, book vendor and teaching material sites, association and center sites, and radiology patient sites.

The appendices include the American College of Radiology standards on both digital image data management and teleradiology, both documents reprinted with the gracious permission of the ACR. The last component of the appendix is the glossary, included to help the reader navigate specific terminology introduced and used throughout the book, and terms associated with computers and the Internet in general.

The purpose of this text is to help all radiologists and radiology personnel at any level of computer expertise understand and harness the powers of the Internet. For those who have relatively little experience with the Internet, this book can help them come up to speed. For those with a moderate level of experience, it is meant to provide resources and factual data that will help them get more from the tools that are currently available. And lastly, for the experienced user, it is a reference tool that provides links and references to other locations where information of a higher level can be obtained. This book was written with the radiology practice in mind, but the ubiquity of the Internet and its related technologies applies to all in the health care field.

One final point: It always is of utility to learn from the experience of others. Thus, in appropriate areas of the text, we have used real-life examples from our experiences at the Massachusetts General Hospital of the Harvard Medical School. These experiences are not meant to serve as guidelines of how to implement technologies, but as examples in order to understand potential pitfalls.

It is my sincere hope that you will find this text useful in your day-to-day activities.

I
Background

1
The Internet/World Wide Web (WWW)

The Concepts

A Very Brief History

The Internet was first implemented in the late 1960s as a United States Department of Defense initiative called the ARPAnet. The ARPAnet originally was formed primarily to support military research on how to build networks that could withstand outages and continue to function properly in the event a single connection or location on the network was rendered out of commission. The network design approach assumed that the network itself was not unreliable, which is a very realistic approach if one considers the stability in the design of these computer elements and barring an act of nature or a bomb attack. Since the original ARPAnet model mandated that all communications occur between two computers directly, any segment of the network could suffer downtime, but communication between the other computers on the network would still continue via alternate routes across the network. What was needed for two computers to communicate was a message that was enclosed in a standard format, which was then and still is called the Internet Protocol (IP) packet, along with the address of the destination computer.

As the network was put in place and was found to be quite robust in its operation, continual upgrades were made. In the early 1980s, the advent of the Ethernet brought about faster networks and the concept of local area networks (LANs). At this time, however, most of the computers on LANs were still UNIX-based workstations. These workstations came with built-in IP networking capabilities, since these computers were often destined for large-scale applications such as the military. The organizations that were purchasing these computers wanted to connect their machines to the ARPAnet. As all the nodes on the network were using the IP "language," it became obvious that there were benefits in enabling users on one network to communicate with those on any other network or LAN.

In the late 1980s, the National Science Foundation (NSF) created five supercomputer centers around the country. These computers were meant to serve academic research centers around the country, since costs were prohibitive to install these machines in each major academic center. At the time, the ARPAnet seemed to be the ideal solution to this communication problem, but, due to political reasons, this plan was never undertaken. As an alternate solution, the NSF took the network building knowledge of the ARPAnet and built its own network, named the NSFNET, with connections running over special telephone lines at 56 kilobytes per second (kbps). Although these lines are slow by today's standards, they were prohibitively expensive. Since the telephone companies were charging by the mile, it was in the interest of the NSF to create regional networks, allowing sites to connect to the nearest next user, in a "daisy-chain" fashion. Each daisy chain then could be connected to one of the regional supercomputer centers, and all the centers in turn then were linked together.

This network was a great success and soon became overloaded when researchers discovered that it was useful for sharing resources above and beyond the work directly related to the supercomputers. In the late 1980s, an outside firm received a contract to maintain and upgrade the network. Over time, the original NSF network was replaced with telephone lines and computers that were faster. The network was opened to all researchers, government employees, and special contracted agencies. Access was permitted to international organizations and, in the early 1990s, to commercial sites. Over the course of the last decade, this growth has exploded, and the majority of households and businesses have access to the network in some form or another.

What Is the Internet Today and How Does It Affect the Radiologist?

The Internet has been the fastest growing technology of all time; each day brings a new use. You have, without a doubt, already heard about the Internet or used it to gather news, stock quotes, do shopping, search for information, or send gifts, among a myriad of other functions. For the medical community, the Internet represents an ideal mechanism not only for the delivery of care, but also for learning and sharing information. For radiology, the Internet promises to provide solution, such as teleradiology applications, to many day-to-day problems and make available a multitude of other services that impact education and equipment purchase.

Radiologists always have dealt with and will continue to deal with receiving, analyzing, and interpreting data, whether it be in the form of images or text. The relay of this information to the source, whether it be a patient or referring physician, has been performed via various routes as technology has progressed over the past several decades: via phone, mail, and fax and now via e-mail or the World Wide Web. We have already seen the implementation of many of the concepts of the Internet in our departments with digital-based modalities and the PACS (picture archiving and communication systems). The Internet represents both a means of extending the reach of these tools as well as a way to make them more efficient within our own departments.

The Internet will without a doubt have an impact on both your personal and professional life, and will make it easier. While the majority of the direct functions and resources of the Internet are of a reference nature to most radiologists (e.g., looking up a reference article for an interesting case or creating an on-line teaching file), many of the technologies and functions that have been developed and are continually being refined are technologies that are *enabled* by the Internet. These are technologies that use the concepts of networking and the infrastructure that the Internet has popularized and apply them to functions that make us more efficient as radiologists. Thus, while many of the direct functions and uses of the Internet may not seem of great utility to you currently, once the enabled technologies become more commonplace, the integration of these components will promise to affect the way you practice. It is now a time when many of the technologies are in their infancy and when one can grasp the fundamental concepts. If these are mastered, with the ubiquity of the Internet and its impartiality to geographic location, any individual can begin to create tools and resources from which the rest of the community can benefit.

The Bricks: Networks

To fully use the Internet for its power, one must understand a few basics about networks. In its simplest definition, a network is a group of two or more computers linked together. There are many types of networks and many schemes to describe them. While the specifics of how to connect computers in a network is beyond the scope of what a user needs to understand, a fundamental understanding of how a network works can often aid in understanding why something you are trying to accomplish will not work.

In "network-speak," computers on the network are called *nodes* or clients. There is a special main computer on most networks that allocates the resources for the entire network, and this computer is called a *server*. These two terms thus define the "client-server" model in which there is a central computer designated the server that often provides information or services to the many client computers.

The manner in which the servers and clients on networks are configured is termed the network topology. The most common general network topologies include the bus, star, and ring configurations, which look like what they are called and are diagrammed in Figure 1.1. The star, bus, and ring topologies are just one method used to describe the configuration of a network. There are, however, multiple other schemes that computer professionals use that may come up when describing the network that you may be connecting to from home or from a hospital. The most popular of these network descriptions refer to the distance between computers or networks and are termed local area networks (LANs), metropolitan area networks (MANs), and wide area networks (WANs).

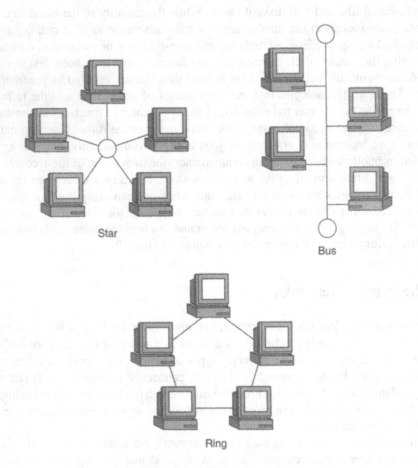

FIGURE 1.1. Various network configurations described by the arrangement of the network.

What Are LANs, WANs, and MANs?

A LAN is a network of connected computers that share the resources of a single processor or server that is within a relatively small geographic area. Often, this is the area of an office or a building. In most radiology departments, the computers in the reading rooms and the radiologists' offices are connected on a LAN, and a suite of application programs are accessible on this network. A WAN possesses the same infrastructure as a LAN, but refers to a network that has a wider geographic reach. The WAN in the radiology department example above would be the hospital network into which the radiology LAN is connected. Lastly, as the name implies, a MAN encompasses an even larger geographic region. A MAN would be the network that connects to another hospital or the entire infrastructure that connects the different facilities in a university medical system.

Other Description Schemes

Another way used to describe a network is by the category of connections between computers (for example, fiber optic, coaxial cable, or copper wire) or the type of communications technology connecting the computers, the most common and popular being the Ethernet. The Ethernet is the most widely used technology in conventional LANs. An Ethernet LAN typically uses coaxial cable (Figure 1-2) or special grades of what are termed twisted pair wires. The twisted pair wires come to an end in an Ethernet jack diagrammed in Figure 1-3. The Ethernet jack will plug into your computer through a network interface card (NIC) (Figure 1-4). The other end connects either to the wall or into a box termed a hub (Figure 1-5) or router that allows multiple computers to connect before then connecting into another connection within the wall.

The most commonly installed Ethernet systems are called 10BASE-T and allow a transmission speed of up to 10 megabits per second (Mbps). In a radiology department, the digital acquisition devices, such as computed tomography (CT) and magnetic resonance imaging (MRI) are connected to a network via Ethernet. As amounts of data transferred over networks begin to increase, especially with newer technology such as multislice CT that can generate upwards of 1,000 images per study, networks need to improve performance through speed. Fast Ethernet or 100BASE-T provides transmission speeds of up to 100 Mbps. Departments are beginning to see the installation of a gigabit Ethernet that provides an even higher level of transmission speed of 1,000 Mbps (1 billion bits per second).

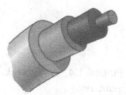

FIGURE 1.2. Diagram of coaxial cable.

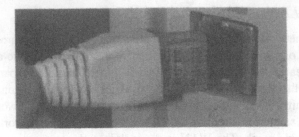

FIGURE 1.3. An Ethernet cable/plug (RJ-45). (Reproduced with permission *www.power-max.com*.)

What Is an Intranet?

Following the widespread availability of Web browsers and servers, many companies realized they could use the same software and protocols that were being used on the Internet at large on their own private internal networks. Using these protocols made sense, as these had been thoroughly tested over the past two decades and had proven to be robust. In addition, using these "standard" protocols meant that the internal networks could easily communicate with the outside world and obviate expensive integration and synchronization efforts. Thus, these internal networks that were shielded from the outside world but could communicate with it were termed "intranets." The Internet thus became the "outside" network and the "intranet" became the internal network.

Thus, an intranet is simply a network that provides a similar function as the Internet to a smaller group, such as a radiology department or a hospital. While

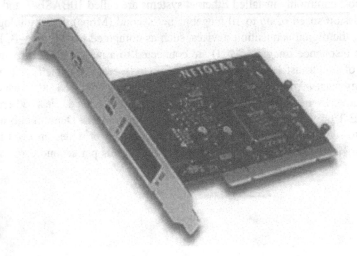

FIGURE 1.4. A network interface card. (Reproduced with permission from *www.net-gear.com*.)

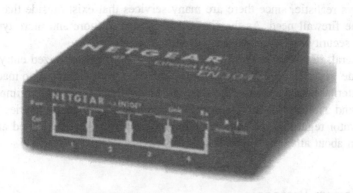

FIGURE 1.5. An Ethernet hub. (Reproduced with permission from *www.netgear.com*.)

in most instances an intranet uses the same protocols and architecture as the Internet, it is not always connected to the Internet. This can be due to security reasons or to the fact that there is no need for certain intranet systems to access the tools and resources of the Internet. For example, an intranet connecting several CT scanners to a printer and a workstation does not need to access the Internet if teleradiology or integration into a PACS is not desired.

What Is a Firewall?

When discussing the concepts of networks, intranets, and the Internet, the issue of security is often raised. With the creation of an intranet, it is the choice of the administrator whether or not to connect the intranet to the Internet. If the decision is made not to connect to the outside world, there is no concern of intruders entering the network due to the absence of connections. However, when the intranet is connected to the outside world, as is often the case in hospitals where users need the resources of Medline, teaching files, and office management or image transmission capabilities, administrators must utilize some form of protection. This protection is termed a "firewall."

A firewall is a system that enforces the access between two networks. The exact technical specifics by which this protection is conferred varies widely, but the concept behind the firewall can be thought of as two mechanisms: one that blocks traffic on the network and another that permits traffic. Thus, with the mechanisms in place, a firewall essentially will keep certain users out of your network while still allowing you to acquire data and information from the network beyond your physical walls.

While the firewall technology sounds like it solves all the security problems of a network, there are certain shortcomings. Robust protection is provided when a network administrator specifies that only certain data can traverse a firewall, for example, only e-mail. In this situation, the network is protected against any attacks other than attacks against the e-mail service. The scenario, however, is not always realistic, since there are many services that exist outside that users within the firewall need. As the firewall is opened to more and more types of data, the security risk is increased.

In general, firewalls are designed to protect against unauthorized entry from the outside world. This primarily prevents intruders from logging onto machines on the internal network within the firewall. Firewalls also provide an important logging and auditing function, since they are able to provide summaries to the administrator regarding the type and amount of traffic that has passed and information about attempts to break in.

The Mortar: Protocols

A protocol is a standard describing how data are transmitted over networks. Essentially, a protocol is a "language." To speak to other individuals, one must speak their language. Similarly, to communicate with other computers on the Internet or within a hospital, your computer must speak the same language. Just as a language acts as a standard to allow people to communicate, these protocols exist to permit computers of different types in different locations to talk to each other. For example, while communicating on the Internet, it makes no difference if the machine you are using is a Macintosh, an IBM PC, or a UNIX workstation. As long as the machine you are using speaks the same "language" or uses the protocols that are commonplace on the Internet, the connection to the other user will be seamless. Thus, these protocols enable the widespread use of the Internet. For the radiologist and radiology personnel, a cursory understanding of a few of these standards is necessary. There are, however, standards that are specific to medicine that serve specific needs within the radiology and medical community. These are explained in the latter portion of this chapter.

General Internet Protocols and Languages

These are protocols that you likely will encounter when setting up your computer or when troubleshooting things that go wrong. Once setup is completed or if problems do not occur, it is unlikely that you will ever have to deal with them again.

TCP/IP

Transmission Control Protocol/Internet Protocol is the most utilized and likely the most important protocol that you will hear about when hooking up your computer to the Internet. TCP/IP is a group of protocols that essentially define how data are sent over the Internet. To communicate over the Internet, your computer has specific instructions that tell it how to speak this protocol; this is usually transparent to you as the user.

SLIP and PPP

Serial Line Internet Protocol and *Point-to-Point Protocol* are other common methods of connecting to the Internet. SLIP is an older and a simpler protocol than PPP, but to the user their function is similar when connecting to the Internet. Usually, the terms SLIP and PPP come into play when certain Internet service providers use one of these protocols. These protocols connect you to the Internet and make you a node on the network. Once established as a node, your computer uses TCP/IP to communicate.

SMTP

The Send Mail to Person protocol is used to transfer e-mail between computers, usually over Ethernet. Most e-mail systems that send mail over the Internet use SMTP to send messages from one e-mail server to another e-mail server. The messages that are housed on that server can then be retrieved with an e-mail application using either the *Post Office Protocol* (POP) or *Internet Message Access Protocol* (IMAP) protocols. While SMTP sends messages from server to server, it also is generally used to send messages from a mail client to a mail server. You will need to specify both the POP or IMAP server and the SMTP server when you set up your e-mail application.

POP

The *Post Office Protocol* is used to retrieve e-mail from a mailserver once it has been sent using SMTP. There are two versions of POP. The first is called *POP2*, which became an e-mail standard in the 1980s. This version of the protocol required SMTP to send messages. The newer *POP3* can be used with or without SMTP. While the majority of e-mail applications use POP, there are, however, some applications that use the newer IMAP or *Internet Message Access Protocol*.

IMAP

The *Internet Message Access Protocol* also is used to retrieve e-mail. The latest version, IMAP4, is similar to POP3; however, it contains some enhancements, such as real-time searching through e-mail messages for words while messages still reside on the mail server. This enables the user to choose which messages to download onto a local computer.

HTTP

HTTP is short for the *Hypertext Transfer Protocol*, which is the underlying protocol used by the World Wide Web. HTTP is a protocol that defines how messages are formatted and transmitted over the Internet for the WWW. It determines what actions Web servers and browsers perform in response to the various commands they receive. For example, when you enter a Web site address into the location field in a browser, you are actually sending an HTTP command to the Web server and instructing it to direct and receive the information requested in the form of the Web page.

HTML

Hypertext Markup Language is the authoring language used to create Web pages on the WWW. HTML essentially tells the computer how to structure and lay out a Web-based document.

XML

Extensible Markup Language was developed by the World Wide Web consortium to enable Web designers to create their own customized tools. These tools enable the definition, transmission, validation, and interpretation of data between applications on the Internet.

Similar issues to using VRML exist with XML, and an XML-capable browser or plug-in is required. This language has great potential in radiology, since it allows radiology programmers the freedom to create truly interconnected image repositories and textual information that can be manipulated on the World Wide Web to create teaching files, continuing medical education (CME) over the Internet, and image databases.

VRML

Virtual Reality Modeling Language is used to display three-dimensional objects on the World Wide Web. VRML essentially is a three-dimensional version of HTML. Since this is a different language from HTML, a VRML-capable browser or a VRML plug-in to an existing Web browser is required to view documents that are written with the VRM language.

The specific use of VRML in radiology is to produce a three-dimensional space that appears on the screen. The user then can move around within this virtual space. This can be of utility in certain areas of work flow in a radiology department, such as selecting virtual reading rooms for modality-specific or subspecialty studies once a department is set up for digital information.

Java

Java is a programming language developed by Sun Microsystems. Java is termed an object-oriented programming language and is similar to many other languages such as C++ (pronounced see-plus-plus).

Documents written in the Java language are interpreted by the Java Virtual Machine. The Java Virtual Machine interpreter resides on the user's computer and is available for every major operating system environment, including UNIX, Macintosh, and Windows.

Because Java is a general-purpose programming language, it contains a set of features that lend it to programming for use on the World Wide Web. Once a small Java application is written, it is called a Java applet, and this applet can be downloaded to the user's computer from a Web server and executed by a Java-compatible Web browser.

Active X

Another protocol that you may encounter if you decide to create web-based teaching files is *Active X*, a loosely defined set of technologies that have been developed by Microsoft. Active X is an outgrowth of two other Microsoft technologies called *OLE* (object linking and embedding) and *COM* (component object model). The term itself is confusing as it applies to a complete set of COM-based technologies. However, in common parlance, most people think only of Active X "controls," which represent a specific way of implementing the Active X technologies.

Health-Care Protocols

The previously described protocols are ones that every individual who uses the Internet will face. There are, however, certain standards and protocols specific to the health care industry that define objects and their relationships. These protocols are essentially layers on top of existing communication methods and ensure the maintenance of predefined standards. They are discussed below.

HL-7 (Health Level 7)

HL-7 was founded in 1987 to develop a standard for the electronic interchange of primarily clinical, but also financial and administrative, information. This communication occurred primarily on health care oriented computer systems, including hospital information systems, laboratory systems, and pharmacy systems.

The HL-7 standard is supported by almost all vendors of health care computer systems and is used in most U.S. hospitals today. It also is used in Australia, Austria, Germany, Holland, Israel, Japan, New Zealand, and the United Kingdom.

HL-7 essentially standardizes and allows communication between health care devices dealing with patient data. For the radiologist, HL-7 comes into play when integrating the radiology information system (RIS) with the hospital information system (HIS). Since the RIS is an integral component of the PACS, a properly functioning RIS-HIS interface ensures that the reports generated by the radiologist that reside on the RIS are transported over to the HIS and are available to the health care enterprise in a timely fashion.

DICOM (Digital Imaging Communications in Medicine) v3.0 Standard

This standard helps define certain conformance issues between radiology devices. In the past several years, this has expanded to encompass other specialties, including interventional cardiology and dermatology; however, the initial standard was created with radiologic imaging in mind.

DICOM compliance guarantees that acquisition, communication, or display devices will be compliant with all other types of similar devices. The DICOM standard originated from a joint committee that was formed consisting of users, represented by the American College of Radiology (ACR), and medical imaging equipment vendors, represented by the National Electrical Manufacturers Association (NEMA). This committee produced a series of standards beginning with ACR-NEMA 1.0 in 1985, which was later revised, becoming the ACR-NEMA 2.0 standard released in 1989. These older standards were not adopted by many radiology device vendors, since digital imaging and the need for a standard was not essential. What this meant for the radiology department trying to go digital was that many devices were outputting image data in a format that no other piece of hardware on the system could understand. For a short period while digital imaging was becoming popular and vendors were not making their hardware DICOM compliant, smaller companies were able to make a business of making "boxes" that would convert proprietary data from a digital modality—CT, MRI, nuclear medicine or ultrasound (US)—into a DICOM format so that the remainder of the system could store, print, and display these data.

As digital imaging became more commonplace and users began to demand connectivity among their multiple acquisition devices, storage devices, and distribution devices, the earlier ACR-NEMA standards ultimately formed the basis for the now-labeled DICOM 3.0 standard. DICOM compliance for new devices is practically mandated to ensure connectivity into a PACS. As new technology is developed, such as newer compression standards that will improve the quality of teleradiology service, it is incorporated into the DICOM standard after the committee decides whether it will improve the standard of care.

There are other more esoteric health care protocols that usually affect only technology professionals who are involved in health care. The complexity of these protocols is beyond the experience of most radiologists; when events arise involving these protocols, it is the technology professionals who are better suited to solve these problems.

Imaging Standards and Protocols

The previously described protocols are those that are concerned with connectivity from the home or office to the Internet and with the language spoken over these networks by health care equipment. There are still other types of standards that will affect the radiologist. These are used when working with images and define how they are delivered over the Internet and networks, or between computers.

Compression

These standards usually refer to different compression methods utilized to make image files smaller. When an image is captured, there is a large amount of data that make up the image. Within this image, there often are portions that are redundant. By using computer algorithms, redundant portions of image data can be eliminated or compressed. These algorithms or image formats are termed JPEG, GIF, TIFF, etc. Before going into the definition of these compression schemes, a brief understanding of how things are compressed is useful. There are two types of compression: lossy and lossless. These terms become particularly applicable to radiology when one considers the storage of digital images in a digital department. Within a digital department and with the generation of digital images from CT, MR, US, nuclear medicine, and computed radiography, there is a need for large storage devices. As the size of the radiology studies grows, especially with multislice CT and multiple sequences for MRI, techniques must be employed to reduce the size of images without losing the necessary diagnostic information that is contained in those images. Additionally, if images are to be distributed using the Internet, technology to reduce the size of transmitted data and to decrease transmission time becomes a necessity.

Lossy vs. Lossless

Compression can be accomplished via two methods: lossy or lossless. Generally, lossless compression is accomplished using a method by which all data are preserved, and lossy compression is accomplished using a method by which some data are lost, but essentially all clinically relevant data are preserved.

An example of how lossless compression operates is as follows: if the number set 7777 6666 1111 0000 is lossless compressed, it will be stored as 74 64 14 04, which, with the appropriate decompression algorithm (software package), will expand and display 7777 6666 1111 0000. In this particular example, the compression algorithm, without losing any data, has been able to reduce 16 bytes to 8 bytes. With a 2-to-1 compression ratio, all data are preserved within one-half the storage space. Alternatively, an example how lossy compression works is as follows: when the same number set, 7777 6666 1111 0000, is compressed using a lossy method, it will be stored as 78 18, which closely approximates the original data set. Thus, when expanded and displayed again with an appropriate decompression algorithm, the following will be displayed: 7777 7777 1111 1111. A reduction from 16 bytes to 4 bytes is achieved, representing a 4-to-1 compression ratio. In this situation, however, there is a loss of the integrity of the original data, which in certain instances is inconsequential. Within radiology, however, it is questionable if it is clinically irrelevant. This method ultimately serves to employ only one-fourth of the storage space of the original data. With the average radiology examination using 20 megabytes (MB) of storage space, lossless compression results in each exam using less than 10 MB of storage space. Utilizing lossy compression, such as wavelet algorithms, the same study, with a 20:1 compression ratio, will use just greater than 1 MB per exam.

Various image compression algorithms use lossy or lossless schemes. The radiologist should know which algorithm is being used because, if images are lossy compressed, one will be aware that a certain amount of the original data is lost. Whether these data are critical to interpretation and diagnosis is at the discretion of the receiving radiologist. Thus, prior to implementation of a teleradiology system, it is often of utility to look at several compression algorithms and decide which are of diagnostic quality to the particular observer. Below is a list of common image compression algorithms.

JPEG

The Joint Photographic Experts Group standard was the work of a group of experts nominated by national standards bodies and major companies to work together and create a compression mechanism that could be adopted widely. JPEG is designed for compressing either full-color or gray-scale images of natural, real-world scenes. The standard works well on photographs, naturalistic artwork, and similar material, but not as well on lettering or complex line drawings. The JPEG standard was created to handle exclusively still images, but a related standard called MPEG (Motion Picture Expert Group) exists for movie formats.

JPEG is a lossy compression scheme; however, this is usually transparent to most users since the JPEG mechanism is designed to exploit known limitations of the human eye: most notably, small color changes are perceived less accurately than small changes in brightness. Within radiology, a useful property of JPEG is that the degree of lossiness can be varied by adjusting compression parameters. What this allows users to do is change the compression setting so that the quality of the image is improved at a lesser compression ratio.

As a radiologist, you may see many of the images of radiographs, CTs, MRIs, etc., that you download from the Internet in the form of teaching files or case reports in the JPEG format. As image compression technology matures and the speed with which computers can compress and decompress data increases, newer standards are being developed. Over the last several years, we have seen the

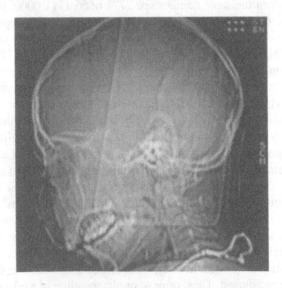

FIGURE 1.6. Original image uncompressed.

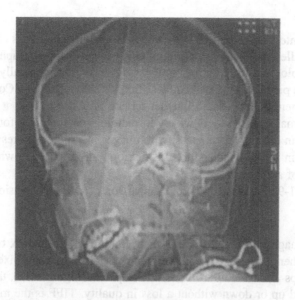

FIGURE 1.7. Original image compressed with JPEG at 34:1 with a size savings of 71.3%. Note the loss of clarity of the skull.

growth and popularity of the JPEG2000 standard. This standard is an extension of the JPEG format described above, but promises improved compression and retention of image data.

See Figures 1-6, 1-7, and 1-8 for comparison of various JPEG compression levels.

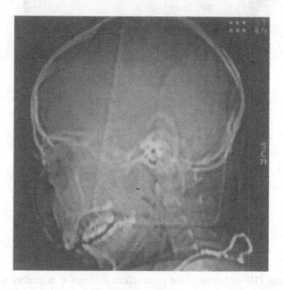

FIGURE 1.8. Original image compressed with JPEG at 52:1 with a size savings of 81.0%. Note the loss of clarity of the facial bones.

GIF

The Graphics Interchange Format is a standard for digitized images compressed with what is called the "LZW" algorithm. GIF is a bit-mapped graphics format and supports color and different resolutions. However, it is generally better for black and white pictures. This standard was first defined in 1987 by CompuServe (CIS), a prominent bulletin board/Internet service provider.

The GIF format is not used as widely in radiology as the other formats. It is primarily used in creating Web pages, with images in which compression is utilized to make an image smaller for transmission, and in cases in which image quality is less of a concern.

See Figures 1-9, 1-10, and 1-11 for comparison of GIF compression levels.

TIFF

The Tagged Image File Format is a bitmap graphic file format. A bitmap is a graphic that, when magnified, is composed of dots (also known as pixels or bits). Because bitmaps are made up of thousands of pixels (Figure 1-12), they cannot easily be scaled up or down without a loss in quality. TIFF is the most widely used bitmap graphic format in the printing world.

Wavelet

Wavelet compression is a lossy compression technique that is based on a mathematical algorithm. The mathematics behind wavelet compression are complex;

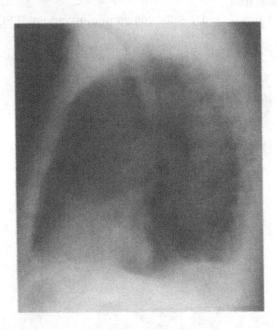

FIGURE 1.9. Original GIF of lateral chest x-ray. Note difference in quality when compared to prior JPEG images.

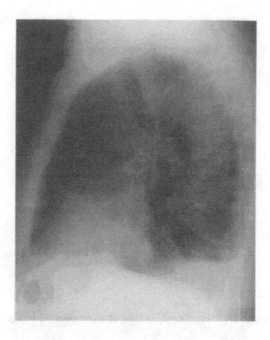

FIGURE 1.10. Compressed GIF by 41.7%. Note the degradation of quality.

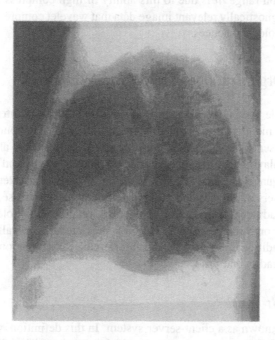

FIGURE 1.11. Compressed GIF by 86.1%. Note the image is uninterpretable.

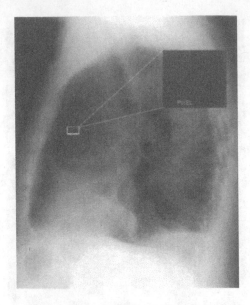

FIGURE 1.12. Pixel composition of a compressed image.

however, from the user's perspective, wavelet compression allows reductions in the size of an image without significant degradation in diagnostic quality into the 30:1 compression range. It is due to this ability of high compression ratios with retention of diagnostically relevant image data that wavelet compression is widely used in teleradiology practices.

Buildings/Organizations: The World Wide Web

The World Wide Web (WWW) is most likely the part of the Internet you have seen frequently mentioned in the media and may have used in your hospital. The WWW to the user is the "graphical" portion of the Internet that allows communication by displaying text, graphics, animation, photos, sound, and video through the HTML language. Because the WWW is a graphic-based system, it is widely popular with users of all ages and all levels of computer expertise, whether they be children or adults, advertisers or consumers, retailers or wholesalers, magazine publishers or resource sites. The WWW has created a parallel medium to many of the traditional advertising and information dissemination mechanisms, including TV, radio, and print.

How Does It Work?

The WWW is known as a client-server system. In this definition, your computer is the client and the remote computer to which you connect is called the server. See Figure 1-13 for a diagram of the client-server relationship.

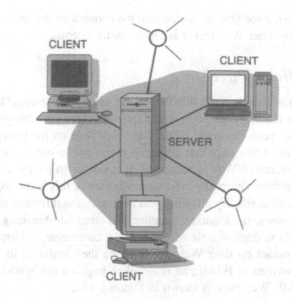

FIGURE 1.13. Diagram of the client-server relationship.

The server in turn is a client for another computer that acts as a server, and, in this daisy-chain fashion, all the computers are connected onto the main backbone of the Internet. By this disseminated architecture, literally millions of computers can become connected and share information through the Web-like network.

The method by which data on the internet/WWW is linked is termed hypertext and hyperlinks. These terms describe the processes that allow electronic files on the WWW to be linked together so that you can navigate through pages of information. A browser (Chapter 3) is used to navigate the hyperlinks contained on Web pages.

What Is a Web Page and a Web Site?

A Web page is an electronic document written in HTML. On the Internet, each Web page has a unique address, called the Uniform Resource Locator (URL), which identifies its location. A group of Web pages is called a Web site. The Web page is the basic building block of each Web site.

Web pages on a Web site are linked together through hyperlinks as described above. Clicking on a link on a page allows you to jump between other pages on a Website and gather the information you need. The collection of Web pages that make up a Web site resides on a Web server, which is a computer designated to house Web sites and is always connected to the Internet. When you ask, through your Web browser, to see specific information on a Web site or Web server, this information is sent over the network to the Web server, which in theory will send you this information. Various Web pages on a Web site may, through hyperlinks, be linked to other Web pages on other Web sites, which are housed on other Web servers; however, once you are linked into the network of the Internet, the electronic trip to the other Web server is almost instantaneous.

What Is a Home Page?

After you have browsed on the WWW you will often see the term "home page." The home page is simply the point on the Internet where you always start. It can be thought of as your electronic home. Any Web page on the Internet can be a home page. It is on this page that information you use to begin linking to other pages on the Internet/WWW is contained. It is similar to a table of contents in a book. Many services currently offer customization of this home page to reflect your interests and needs. By allowing you to display the information relevant to you, including news, stock quotes, weather, and other late-breaking news, these services are able to display their advertising in a concurrent fashion. This home page usually resides on their Web server where they maintain its integrity. A home page is written in HTML, as is any Web page on the World Wide Web. A sample HTML Web page is shown in Figure 1-14.

What Is a URL (Uniform Resource Locator)?

At its core, the WWW is a network of electronic files stored on computers all around the world. The hypertext links connect these resources. The URLs are the addresses used to locate these files. The URL contains the necessary information to jump from one Web page to another with just one click.
What does a typical URL look like? Here are some examples:

http://www.thedigitaldepartment.com—the home page for The Digital Department Web site.

```
<body background="_themes/travel/tratilea.jpg" bgcolor="#003399" text="#FFFFCC"
link="#FFCC00" vlink="#669900" alink="#FFCC00"><!--msnavigation--><table
border="0" cellpadding="0" cellspacing="0" width="100%"><tr><td><!--mstheme--
><font face="times new roman, times">

<p> </p>

<h6><!--mstheme--><font face="impact, arial, helvetica" color="#CCFF00"><img
src="_derived/index.htm_cmp_travel110_bnr.gif" width="600" height="60" border="0"
alt="Rad Exam Info"> <br>
<!--mstheme--></font></h6>

<p> </p>
<!--mstheme--></font></td></tr><!--msnavigation--></table><!--msnavigation--><table
border="0" cellpadding="0" cellspacing="0" width="100%"><tr><td valign="top"
```

FIGURE 1.14. Diagram of sample HTML web page in programming language.

ftp://download.com—a directory of files available for download.
news://sci.med.radiology.intervention—a newsgroup for interventionalists.

The first part of a URL (before the two slashes) illustrates the type of protocol that you are accessing, a Web page if http, a file server for downloading if ftp, a newsgroup if news, etc. The second part of a URL usually is the address of the computer where the data or resource is housed. Specifically, it defines the IP address or the domain name where the resource is located, for example, *www.thedigitaldepartment.com.* Within many URLs there will be a third portion. The third portion, after the single forward slash, usually is the name of a specific Web page written in HTML, hence the .html extension in the following example: *http://www.digitaldepartment.com/home.html.* On most Web browsers, you can enter the URL either by typing it into the "location" window or by going through your "favorites" menu.

A few words on domain name services: As we have previously discussed, the computers on the Internet know where they are on the network by an IP address, which encompasses four sets of numbers separated by periods. It is not practical to expect us to remember all the different numbers for all Web sites and computers. We can, however, remember simple text phrases such as *www.springer-ny.com* for Springer-Verlag in New York. Behind the scenes, each time you enter a Web address, the textual information is converted by a domain name system (DNS) server into a numerical IP address, such as 216.34.122.81, allowing for easier Internet use. Domain names are assigned based on the type of group or site that requests the name. The site type is generally differentiated by the three-letter suffix at the end of the URL. Some of the more common suffixes are .com for commercial sites, .org for nonprofit organizations, and .gov for the government. The countries outside the United States generally use different site-naming conventions. With this knowledge, understand that if you get a DNS error message, it usually means that the DNS server cannot find a specific IP address that matches the name you typed.

What Are Search Engines?

There are millions of Web sites and Web pages on the WWW/Internet. Unless you know the specific location of the information you need, it can be very difficult to navigate and find it. A search engine is a computer program that sits behind a Web site, contains information on the millions of Web sites on the WWW, and has them cataloged in such a way that allows you to search for them. There are a multitude of search engines available to the user, and as the Internet continues to grow there have emerged intelligent search engines that not only will search other search engines, but also will attempt to understand what exactly you are looking for by using artificial intelligence or by analyzing the words and the way they fit together. A search engine is usually the best place to start when you are looking for information. Each search engine catalogs and categorizes the information that it houses in its database in a different way, so searching for the same topic on multiple search engines often yields different results.

How Do They Work?

Typically, a search engine constantly sends out a "spider," which is a program that automatically fetches Web pages. Spiders are used to then, in turn, feed pages back to the specific search engine that sent out the query. The program is called a spider, since it crawls through the WWW. Some computer gurus also refer to spiders as Web crawlers.

Since the Internet grows exponentially on a daily basis, one would imagine that it would be difficult for spiders and search engines to keep up with the growth. Interestingly, because most Web pages contain links to other pages, a spider can start anywhere and constantly search. Immediately following the detection of a link to another page, the spider will fetch it. The larger search engines often have many spiders working in parallel.

As a spider fetches Web pages and sends the information back to the search engine, another program, called an *indexer*, reads these documents and creates an index based on the words contained in the found documents. Each search engine uses its own rules and regulations to create these indexes so that it is able to return the information you request in a useful manner.

If you are thinking of setting up a Web site on a Web server and you want to ensure that as many people as possible are able to reach your site, it is important to submit the information about your Web site to these search engines or have this information solicited.

There are currently many search engines available to users. Each of these search engines uses a slightly different method to catalog and organize information as well as to search through the database in order to return the necessary information that the user requests. For example, a common search engine is *www.Yahoo.com*. This search engine allows the user to enter a word that is then matched against the database; Web pages that its spider has crawled through are displayed. Another engine, *www.Google.com*, uses large-scale data mining and a proprietary technology called "PageRank." PageRank is a patent-pending software package that uses the objective measure of the importance of Web pages by solving an equation of 500 million variables and 2 billion terms. Other search engines include *www.Hotbot.com*, *www.AltaVista.com*, *www.Lycos.com*, and *www.NorthernLight.com*, to name just a few.

What Are Portals?

A portal is defined in the Webster's dictionary as "a doorway, an entrance, or a gate, especially one that is large and imposing." A Web portal is a Web site that is used as an entry point to the Internet. This usually is used as a marketing term, but describes the first place a user would go to when using the WWW. Most portal sites have a catalog of other resources or Web sites and a search engine that will allow you to find other pieces of information. Many of these portal sites now offer other enhanced services, such as e-mail, classifieds, weather, and news, in order to make these sites more appealing to the user. If the portal provides information that is specific to you as a user, it often can organize a great deal of relevant information in a small amount of space and save you the time of having to search the Internet for this information. These Web sites also can charge advertisers for space on their portal main page based on the fact that they have so many users accessing them on a daily basis. Within radiology, there are many portals emerging, some of which are listed in Chapter 9. These radiology portals bring you up-to-date on a daily basis by providing news in radiology, teaching files, and advertising from radiology vendors, among other things.

2
Getting Wired

Computers: Selecting a Computer for the Radiologist

The configurations for personal computers available today are mind-boggling. You can pick everything from the color of the keys on your keyboard to wattage on your subwoofer. Given that there are so many choices, what makes sense for a radiologist who would like to perform more image-intensive data retrieval than the common user? What configuration is required to perform the common tasks of a radiologist, including teleradiology, review of teaching files, report generation through voice recognition, and retrieval of information from the Internet through e-mail, Medline, and other news sources?

The first decision that needs to be made is whether you need an IBM-compatible PC, an Apple Macintosh, or another operating-based system such as UNIX or LINUX. There are pros and cons to each of these machines, but, essentially, when it comes to obtaining information from the Internet, the type of machine is a moot point since most of the information is provided in a format that all platforms are able to understand.

What you should consider is which computer system is more prevalent in your department. If you need to exchange files with your colleagues, friends, or family, you need to known which type of machines they use. It ultimately will be much easier for you to exchange data with them if you are on the same platform they are using, but this is not to say it is not possible to transfer data across platforms. In addition, you must consider the cost of the machine you are purchasing given that technology goes out-of-date rather rapidly. The machine that you buy today may be out-of-date within a few months in terms of the latest technology; however it most likely will be able to serve your needs for a number of years. My advice when purchasing a computer is to buy as much technology as you can within your price range and add upgrades to it as hard drives get bigger and RAM gets cheaper.

Once you have made the decision to purchase a computer on a certain platform, the next decision is what configuration do you need. If the number of microdecisions you have to make when purchasing a computer baffles you, gain solace from the fact that almost every computer available on the market today will serve more than 90% of your needs as a radiologist, so it is almost impossible to purchase the "wrong" computer. There are small configuration differences that will improve your performance.

Central Processing Unit (CPU)

In general, try to purchase as fast a CPU as you can within your budget. This is not to say that the faster the CPU, the faster the computer will be. There are other factors, including bus speed and RAM size and speed to name a few, that ultimately affect the performance of your computer. However, in general, the faster the CPU, the faster the computer you purchase. Why purchase a fast CPU? This will help in two major areas: first, with image-intensive manipulation, such as when dealing with teaching files and teleradiology, things will move a little faster if you have a faster CPU; second, applications such as voice recognition for dictating your reports require higher levels of power in order to operate efficiently.

Random Access Memory (RAM)

You will need to purchase at least 64 megabytes of RAM because many of the teleradiology applications require 64-megabytes as a minimum. You will realize improved performance if you increase this amount to 128 megabytes. Voice recognition software packages will run more smoothly if you have more megabytes of RAM, and you can run more applications simultaneously with this increased amount.

Video Cards/Monitor

Video cards and monitors are usually defined by the resolution of pixels they can output and display, respectively. In general, you will need to purchase a video card and a monitor that are capable of providing and displaying a resolution of at least 1,024 pixels by 768 pixels (conventionally termed 1K × 1K). Most video cards on the market today provide resolutions much higher than this, into the 1,920 × 1,440 range. With the 1K × 1K resolution, most radiologic studies will appear as they do on PACS workstation monitors in the hospital. This will allow you to review both plain film and digital modalities without a great deal of image degradation. The size of the monitor you wish to purchase depends both on your budget and on your personal preference; monitor sizes range from 15" to over 21". In general, larger monitors are desirable, and these have become affordable. Other monitor formats you will encounter, usually in the radiology departments, are 2,048 pixels × 1,760 pixels, or 2K × 2K monitors. These monitors traditionally are used for interpretation of chest x-rays and plain radiographs due to their inherent better resolution. Work on resolution thresholds by Boland demonstrated that 2K monitors are required to detect subtle pneumothoracies. More recent work by our group (Mehta, Boland, and Mueller, 2000) presented at RSNA 2000 demonstrated that 1K monitors are sufficient for plain film abdominal radiography and intravenous pyelogram (IVP) studies.

Other Storage Devices

Today, all computer systems come equipped with CD-ROM drives, and this will be a necessary component for you if you decide to purchase teaching files or CD-ROMs containing textbooks. CD-ROM drives are available in various speeds, starting at 2× and going to 48× and beyond. You should try to purchase the fastest one within reason, given the configuration of your computer. In the same category as CD-ROM drives, computer manufacturers now offer DVD drives to view DVD movies and other titles that come in this format. Some data are now being stored in DVD format instead of on several CD-ROM disks. The choice to purchase a DVD drive depends on the foreseeable use of the computer system in your home or office and whether this is an application that interests you. Some users, however, will find utility in purchasing a CD recordable or CDR device. This allows you to "burn" or make your own CD-ROM disks. This can be useful not only for making teaching files or storing images from cases, but also for more conventional home uses, such as backing up hard drives or creating digital photo albums.

One of the final decisions you have to make is the size of the hard drive. Generally, most computers are equipped with hard drives within the tens to hundreds of gigabyte range, so, once again, you need to gauge what your needs will be. If you plan to store a large number of images on your hard drive, then you should purchase the relative amount of hard drive space for the types of images that you plan to store. For most users, a hard drive in the tens of gigabyte range will provide adequate long-term storage. Table 2-1 lists the sizes of common radiologic studies.

TABLE 2.1. Common sizes for radiologic studies.

Modality	Image matrix	No. of studies	Image file size (Mb)
Mammography	4,096 × 5,120 × 12	4	125.0
Plain radiographs	2,048 × 2,048 × 12	4	25.0
Fluoroscopy	1,024 × 1,024 × 8	18	19.0
Computed tomography (CT)	512 × 512 × 12	30	12.0
Magnetic Resonance Imaging (MRI)	256 × 256 = 12	100	10.0
Ultrasound (US)	256 × 256 × 8	24	1.5
Nuclear medicine	128 × 128 × 8	24	0.4

Connections: What Should I Get?

Once you have purchased your computer or if you already have one, you will need to connect it somehow to the outside world, namely to the Internet. There are essentially two places where you have to consider connecting your computer: at home and within the radiology department. In most instances, there will be an information systems (IS) department within your radiology department. It will be responsible for connecting you to a LAN that will allow you to gather information from the HIS and the PACS and for connecting you to the Internet. But how do you hook up your home computer? There are several options you need to consider when gaining Internet access at home.

POTS: Plain Old Telephone System

The simplest way to gain access to the Internet is over your regular telephone lines. To connect to the Internet in this manner, you will need a modem within, or connected to, your computer. Most computer systems are equipped with a built-in modem, but, at a minimum, you should try to purchase a 56,000 kilobits per second (kbps) modem. Other modem speeds include, historically, 300 kbps, 1,200 kbps, 2,400 kbps, and 9,600 kbps, and, although difficult to find, one can still purchase modems that are 14,400 kbps and 28,800 kbps. See Figure 2-1 for a comparison of download speeds for various dial-up connections.

Once you have your modem, you will need what is called an Internet service provider (ISP). An ISP does exactly what it says: it provides you with a hookup onto the Internet. See Figure 2-2 for a diagram depicting the configuration between your computer and the internet servers. These companies main-

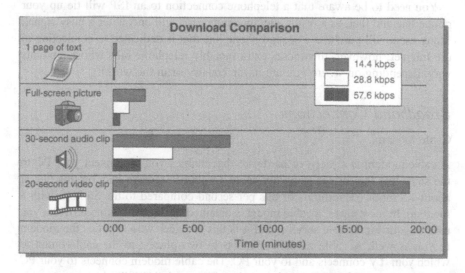

FIGURE 2.1. Comparison of download speeds for various dial-up connections.

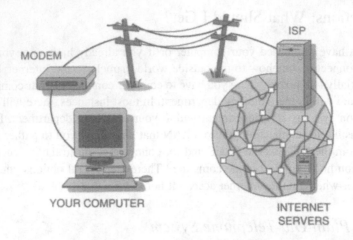

FIGURE 2.2. Schematic representation of the configuration between your computer and Internet servers.

tain large computers with fast connections to portions of the backbone of the Internet and allow you to plug your computer into theirs in order to get onto the highway. Most ISPs have an "all-you-can-use package" for a monthly fee, and others offer a certain number of hours per month. Common ISPs include America Online, Earthlink, and Mindspring. With this method of connection, you need to call into your ISP and negotiate a connection between your computer and theirs each time you need to use the Internet or e-mail. Generally, if you are obtaining news information, stock quotes, and other basic information on the Internet, this type of connection will meet your needs adequately in most instances.

You need to be aware that a telephone connection to an ISP will tie up your phone line and that, as a result, any incoming calls will encounter a busy signal. Many users will purchase a second phone line that is dedicated to connecting to the Internet; however, this incurs extra monthly telephone bills whose amounts vary, depending on where you are in the country or in the world.

Broadband Connections

Cable Modem

A cable modem is a piece of hardware that enables you to connect your PC to the same line that brings you your cable TV and to receive data on this line at about 1.5 mbps (or millions of bits per second compared to the 56 kbps with a modem). In most cases, a cable model is obtained through the same provider you use for your local cable service, and it is this provider who supplies the modem to you as well. A cable modem connects to two places: to the cable outlet to which your TV connects and to your PC. The cable modem connects to your PC via an "Ethernet Card" or "Network interface card (NIC)," which most cable companies will provide to you at a fee or which you can purchase on your own. See Figure 2-3 for a diagram of a cable modem connection.

In contrast to connecting to an ISP with your modem, where all data are sent through your ISP, all cable modems attach via the cable coaxial line to a cable modem termination system (CMTS) at the local cable TV company office. Through this CMTS, the cable modem can receive and send data from the Internet.

Cable companies may tell you that the bandwidth for Internet service over their service is up to 27 mbps on the download path, with somewhere in the range of 2.5 mbps of bandwidth for the upload path. The actual bandwidth that you obtain, once connected, depends ultimately on whether the provider itself is connected to the Internet on a line faster than a T1 at 1.5 mbps. The added benefit of a cable modem, however, in addition to the faster data rate, is that it is a continuous connection that does not require tying up a phone line or calling into an ISP in order to obtain access to the Internet.

Digital Subscriber Line (DSL)

DSL is another high-speed technology that connects you to the Internet. DSL lines can always be connected to the Internet, like cable modems. On most ADSL lines, data can be transferred at rates of up to 1.5 mbps while downloading, as with cable modems, and at about 128 kbps when uploading. ADSL, however, operates over conventional phone lines. The ADSL modem will communicate with the telephone company's Internet provider systems on a portion of the phone line, and your phone still can send along signals simultaneously. As with a cable model, DSL service requires a special modem. See Figure 2-4 for a diagram of a DSL system.

You may hear the term xDSL when you are considering various connection options for your home PC. This term simply refers to different variations of DSL, such as HDSL (high data rate subscriber line) or SDSL (symmetric digital subscriber line). Each of these configurations allows various speeds of uploading and downloading. DSL service may not be offered in all geographic areas due

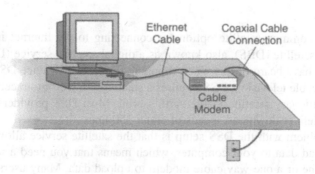

FIGURE 2.3. Sample setup of a cable modem.

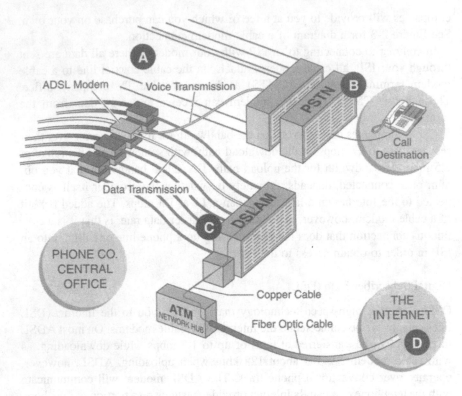

FIGURE 2.4. Schematic representation of a setup of a DSL system.

to restrictions on the distance from the exchange hub or telephone company, usually set at 3 miles. These configurations are continuously evolving, however, and it is best to check with your local phone company to see if DSL is offered in your area.

Less Common Options

Satellite

The most common satellite option for connecting to the Internet is the direct broadcast satellite (DBS), also known as a digital satellite service (DSS). Many users may have heard of this when shopping for cable TV, since DSS is a competitor to cable television. DSS requires a small satellite dish to receive data sent from a stationary satellite in the earth's orbit. Most DSS providers claim that they can deliver download speeds of about 350 kbps.

The problem with the DSS setup is that the satellite service allows you only to download data to your computer, which means that you need a modem with a phone line or a one-way cable modem to upload data. Many users will report that satellite Internet service is usually quite slow because a request for information needs to be sent from your computer over your phone line to the DSS provider, then to the satellite, and then back down to you. The costs for satellite service also vary from provider to provider.

Integrated Services Digital Network (ISDN)

ISDN gained popularity before the cable modem and ADSL became widely available. ISDN offers an intermediate solution in terms of speed that is in between analog modems and cable or DSL. In some areas, cable modem or DSL may not be offered, and ISDN may serve your needs. ISDN works over the standard copper phone wiring and operates at speeds of up to 128 kbps (two 56.6 kbps connections). To use ISDN, you also will need a special modem and an ISP that can support its use.

T1

A T1 line is a dedicated phone connection that supports data rates of up to 1.544 mbits per second. A T1 line consists of 24 individual channels, each of which can carry 64 kbits per second. Each 64 kbit/second channel can be configured individually to carry either data or voice information, and telephone companies often will allow you to buy a section of these channels, this option is known as *fractional T1* access.

T1 lines are generally expensive to use, and usually are leased by large businesses connecting to the Internet and by Internet service providers (ISPs) that provide service to your home for their connection to the Internet backbone. Hospitals often have a T1 connection that will connect them either to the Internet backbone or to another hospital. Although it is not commonly used, T1 lines are sometimes referred to as DS1 lines.

The Internet backbone itself, however, consists of a faster type of connection titled a T3 connection.

T3

A T3 line, much like a T1 line, is a dedicated line that supports data rates of about 43 mbps. A T3 line consists of 672 individual channels, each of which supports 64 kbps.

While the prices of these data lines continue to drop, most T3 lines are used mainly by Internet service providers (ISPs) connecting to the Internet backbone and by the backbone itself. Large hospital and HMO groups may use a T3 connection to connect hospital networks, especially if they are using an electronic medical record or a PACS that spans more than one hospital.

T3 lines are sometimes referred to as DS3 lines.

Other Data Technologies

Asynchronous Transfer Mode (ATM)

ATM is a fast, switching, and scalable bandwidth network methodology that ultimately provides 155 mbps to 644 mbps transmission rates over fiber regular network systems. It is a method used to increase the efficiency of transferring data over the network.

Optical Carrier 3 (OC-3)

OC-3 represents a very high speed service that is primarily utilized by large established ISPs. OC-3 service transmits data at 120 mbps, which is equivalent to three DS3 lines.

Typically, OC-3 service to the user is provided via a telephone company. In some instances, an OC-3 line may be used to connect two hospitals within a group system.

Optical Carrier 12 (OC-12)

This is a further extension of the OC-3 technology, offering speeds of up to four times OC-3 connections or 12 times T3 connections.

Security

While being on the Internet as a continually connected node has benefits, there also are issues with security. As a node on the network that is continually connected, your computer becomes susceptible to attacks and breaches of security. In the dial-up scenario, while technically you are susceptible to an attack, there is less chance of this occurring since the time you are connected to the Internet is limited. Since this is a recognized issue, many solutions have emerged. The most prominent of these is the creation of a firewall (discussed earlier), which protects you from the outside world, but lets you obtain information. You can configure a firewall to be as stringent or as lenient as you desire. Firewalls are available as software packages that are continuously running in the background or are built into hubs or routers (previously discussed). You should be sure, if you choose a continuous connection, that your ISP provide you with some guidance in terms of the appropriate security solution for your needs.

Computer viruses are a constant worry for any computer user. The utilization of firewalls and other protection schemes does not eliminate the need for some method of software virus protection. Although firewalls will protect from uninvited intruders, any data that you do allow in in the form of e-mail, downloads, messages, etc., can always contain computer viruses.

Part II
Tools of Utility

3
General Applications Every Radiologist Will Use

E-mail
  Terminology
  Programs and Applications
  Text and Attachments
  Mailing Lists and Newsgroups

World Wide Web Browsers and Web Skills
  Specific Applications on Browsers
  Medline

E-mail

Electronic mail (E-mail) represents one of the most efficient means of communication between individuals ever devised. The delivery of messages is nearly instantaneous and creates little waste. You can choose to read your e-mail whenever it is convenient, and you can go through a large number of messages in a relatively shorter period of time than it would take to open paper envelopes.

As radiologists, we are able to communicate with colleagues and patients not only in a text format over the Internet via e-mail, but also with images and figures as well. Most radiologists who use e-mail never have trouble understanding why it is much more efficient than mail, fax, or phone for transmitting data.

E-mail allows the sending of messages to a single user, such as a referring physician, multiple users, such as a health care team, or all users on a LAN, such as a hospital. The messages received can be deleted or forwarded to other individuals. With access to electronic mail, one can subscribe to mailing lists in order to receive information on a daily, weekly, or monthly basis.

Electronic mail is different from other Internet services in that the sending and receiving computers do not need to be directly connected with each other while the mail is being delivered. Your incoming e-mail messages are delivered to the server that houses your e-mail and then downloaded to your computer. Your outgoing e-mail messages are created on your computer and then sent to a mail server, which is like a post office. This mail server will determine the best method to use so that the message will reach the intended recipient, this message then is sent on to the next mail server or post office, and this process is repeated until the message reaches the mail server closest to the recipient. This entire process takes from seconds to minutes. One can do anything with e-mail that can be done with regular postal mail, except mail physical objects.

Terminology

When sending e-mail, you must have the same information you would need when sending normal mail via the post office: the recipient's address. To simplify things in the electronic world, the entire address is condensed into a single line, with the first portion representing the "name" and the second the "address" separated by @. The address portion has two components: the first is the name of the company or service, and the second is an extension describing the first portion. For example, common extensions include .com for company, .gov for government, and .edu for education. A generic example of an e-mail address for John who works at a hospital may be as follows: john@hospital.com, if it is a company, or john@hospital.edu, if it is a hospital that receives its e-mail services through a university or college.

Programs and Applications

There are hundreds of possible programs to manage your e-mail for you. These programs are in two major categories. First, there are those that reside on your PC either at home or at work. These are programs that you can open in your local environment, and they will download e-mail from the mail server onto your local hard drive or storage device. The most popular versions of this type of software include Microsoft's Outlook or Outlook Express, Netscape's Communicator, and Qualcomm's Eudora. Many computers come preloaded with versions of these software packages, and your decision to use them should be based on which you find most useful. The second category of e-mail management software includes those that are Web based and reside on the Internet. They involve accessing the Internet/World Wide Web (WWW) through a browser, typically Microsoft's Internet Explorer or Netscape's Netscape Navigator, and logging onto a Web site that manages your e-mail for you. In this fashion, you can view your e-mail as Web pages. The most popular versions of these WWW-based e-mail services include Hotmail and Yahoo. For further information, you can visit these sites at www.hotmail.com or www.yahoo.com and sign up for free.

Text and Attachments

Over the last decade, e-mail has become more robust and allows the user more flexibility in sending information. In its simplest form, most users send text-based messages to other colleagues, friends, or family (Figure 3-1).

To send a text-based message, simply enter the e-mail address of the intended recipient in the "To" field in the format discussed above. If someone were sending a piece of e-mail to me, he would enter Mehta@helix.mgh.harvard.edu. Many e-mail applications offer the ability to enhance the routing of an e-mail through the carbon copy (CC) and blind carbon copy (BCC) functions. A carbon copy is an exact replica of the message sent to the recipient in which both the original recipient and the CC recipients can read the message and see to whom the mes-

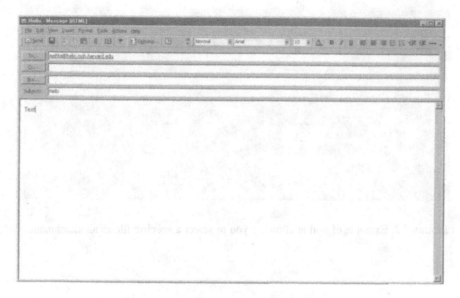

FIGURE 3.1. Text-only e-mail.

sage was sent. This is useful in group committee settings in which you may need to reply to a specific question another committee member has posed, but would like the rest of the group to keep up-to-date with the discussion. The BCC field allows the BCC recipient to read the text of the message, but the original intended recipient of the message does not see who these BCC recipients are, nor is each individual BCC recipient aware of other BCC recipients.

As the popularity of e-mail grew, it became necessary to be able to send other forms of data, namely images and files. Most popular e-mail programs now are able to offer the ability to "attach" documents to an e-mail message. This document then is encoded in a format that can be sent via e-mail and decoded when it arrives at the receiving end. A caveat: some mail servers limit the size of total mail sitting in a mailbox, so if the limit is set at 500K and you send a 1-megabyte image, the mail server will reject the message and send it back to you in its entirety, filling your mailbox with a 1-megabyte file.

To attach a file, such as an image, click on the small paperclip icon found on the message window, in most applications, or on the appropriate menu item to insert or attach a document to your e-mail. This will bring up a pop-up window that will ask you to select the file you would like to attach. If you are sending an image, there usually is an option, in Microsoft Outlook under the insert menu that asks you whether you would like to insert an image and to select its source (Figure 3-2). To see what your final e-mail would look like, see Figure 3-3.

Mailing Lists and Newsgroups

Mailing lists and newsgroups essentially are enhanced e-mail services. They allow you to request e-mail from specialty interest groups, for example, interven-

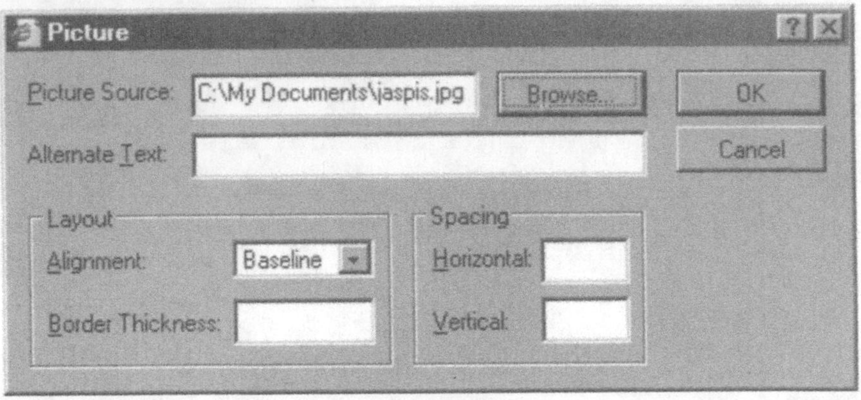

FIGURE 3.2. Example of option allowing you to select a specific file as an attachment.

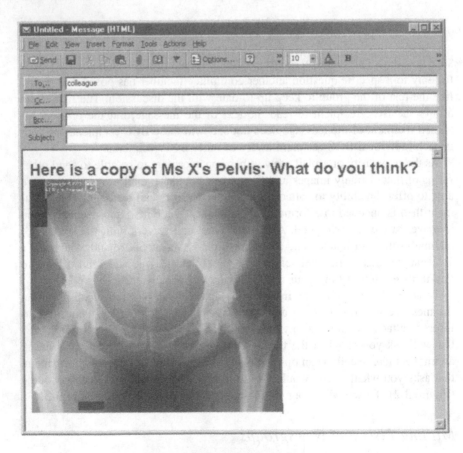

FIGURE 3.3. E-mail with attachment.

tional radiology, or allow you to send mail to a specific group of individuals, for example, European radiologists.

Most mailing lists are set up to forward any message sent to the list to all members of the mailing list. As a user, you subscribe to the electronic mailing list by sending a request in the form of an e-mail message to the list's administrator; usually, this means sending a message with the word "subscribe" in the subject field. Some mailing lists, however, have specific requirements, and you must investigate these prior to joining: for example, the European Forum of Radiologists (EUFORA) requires you to be a radiologist to join.

Newsgroups can be thought of as a worldwide collection of constantly updated bulletin boards, with each pin-up message representing an electronic "post." The difference is that these bulletin boards can be seen by millions of people at the same time without having to wait in line to read the latest message posted on the board. Electronic bulletin boards are very useful for many topics, including consultation, purchasing, and discussion; you will find everything from announcements to in-depth technical discussions regarding the technology of multislice scanners. Articles within each newsgroup are usually arranged into topics. Topics within a newsgroup about musculoskeletal radiology, for example, may include forums on protocols, interesting cases, and consultation. When a post is made to the newsgroup, there are often several responses that will form a "message thread." The software package used to read a newsgroup will decipher and link together those messages that are related. The difference between e-mail and news from a newsgroup is that, when a message is sent to a newsgroup, the message is stored on a news server instead of on your mail server or on your hard drive.

News groups are structured in the form of a hierarchy. Each newsgroup has a name with periods in it qualifying its descriptors. For example, sci.med.radiology.interventional translates into the newsgroup hierarchy SCIENCE MEDICINE RADIOLOGY INTERVENTIONAL. There are several top-level newsgroup categories, including ALT or alternative discussions, BIONET, BIZ, COMP, MISC, and NEWS. There currently are more than 15,000 active newsgroups covering virtually every topic. To connect to a newsgroup, you need a newsgroup reader. Many of the main office packages available on the market include a newsgroup reader. If one is not available, it can be downloaded for free from *www.download.com*. Once you obtain a newsreader, you need the name of the "server" to which you as the "client" can connect. This is provided by your ISP and usually follows the form "news.XXX.com," where XXX represents your ISP. The protocol used is termed the Network News Transfer Protocol (NNTP).

Of note is that newsgroups are not peer-reviewed, and posts can be made anonymously. Thus, information contained within these threads are based on the opinions of the users. Information often can be very selective, incomplete, or incorrect either by omission or by intent. In addition, users can masquerade as physicians or administrators and make posts without the credibility to refute claims. Before posting to a newsgroup, be sure that you are comfortable with making your e-mail address public in this forum or utilize the anonymous post option.

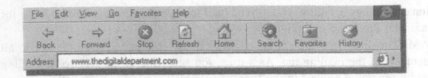

FIGURE 3.4. Internet Explorer.

World Wide Web Browsers and Web Skills

A World Wide Web browser is the software program you use to access the World Wide Web, the graphical portion of the Internet. The first browser, called NCSA Mosaic, was developed at the National Center for Supercomputing Applications in the early 1990s. The easy-to-use point-and-click interface helped popularize the Web, although at that time it was difficult to imagine the immense popularity that the Web would soon enjoy. A Web browser operates by using protocols to request data: for example, a browser or server will send an HTTP request to instruct the receiving Web server to send an HTML encoded Web page. The HTML Web page may include references to other Web documents using *hyperlinks* and other content such as images and audio and visual ("multimedia") content. As the Internet developed over the last decade, many versions of Web browsers were created. Although many different browsers are available, Microsoft Internet Explorer and Netscape Navigator are the two most popular (Figures 3-4 and 3-5). Netscape and Microsoft have invested such great effort in their products that the smaller Web browsers have not been able to maintain the enhancements the users demand. While the basic functionality of the two programs is the same in browsing the WWW, there are many add-on features that appeal to individual users, including integrated e-mail and newsgroups as well as multimedia video and sound players and ease of use.

One of the most important functions of browser software is to help you to request the information that you need. While you can surf for hours on end aimlessly, the Web browser helps you navigate to specific information. Both Netscape Navigator and Internet Explorer come integrated with links to search capabilities as well as resources to link you to places on the Internet that can give you the information you need.

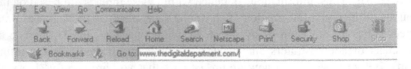

FIGURE 3.5. Netscape Navigator.

Specific Applications on Browsers

Medline

As previously described, there are millions of Web sites providing useful information to the radiologist that can be navigated using a browser on the Internet/WWW. One of the most common reasons physicians use the Internet is for the use of Medline. One of the most utilized sources of Medline information is provided free of charge by the National Library of Medicine through the PUBMED service (Public Medline), which can be reached at *http://www.ncbi. nlm.nih.gov/PubMed/*. By entering this URL into the location bar of your Web browser, you should reach the home page of the PUBMED service.

Once on the home page of this Web site, you can enter key words, authors, or titles of the articles for which you are searching. For a sample of what the home page looks like, see Figure 3-6. The PUBMED service offers a graphic-based query system into the MEDLINE database. It provides the user with the capability to request information about on article.

There are many other interfaces that allow users to query into the MEDLINE database, most of which can be found by doing a search with an Internet search

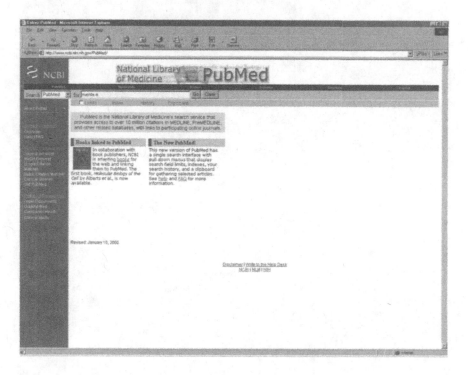

FIGURE 3.6. Sample Web page from the PUBMED search engine.

engine on the keyword "MEDLINE." Some of these Web sites offer various value-added services to entice the physician to use the service.

Once you have obtained the information you requested through the MEDLINE query, this information then can be entered into a database or teaching file or e-mailed to a colleague, since all the information is digital. If you wish to file this information for an upcoming publication, it can be printed, saved to a disk, or burned onto a CD-ROM. The options are endless.

4
Electronic Education: Teaching Files and the Internet

Creating an Internet-Based Teaching File
  Step 1: Obtaining Digital Images
    Converting Analog Film
    Transferring Already-Existing Digital
      Images

Step 2: Adding Textual Data
Step 3: Distribution
Step 4: Viewing Your Teaching File
What About CME?

Teaching film files have been used for many years in teaching normal radiologic anatomy to medical students and residents, and as part of continuing education. The various imaging procedures and the wide spectrum of pathologic conditions that can be diagnosed with radiologic images lend themselves to a case-format collection. However, teaching film collections are cumbersome to manage in terms of storage, retrieval, and sharing with other educators. The advent of the personal computer led to an early revolution by providing a more efficient means of managing educational material. With further advances in CD-ROM technology and especially in the Internet, a great opportunity became available to share radiology teaching collections.

Many radiologists during their careers have developed large collections of interesting cases. These cases have been invaluable for teaching the students who are in close vicinity to these educators; however, they are of limited use to those students in underserviced or remote geographic locations. Progressive educators in the last decade began to develop Internet- and World Wide Web (WWW)-based teaching files. This solution has led to a wider audience and a greater use of interesting case material.

The CD-ROM is a common and attractive format for two reasons: first, the CD-ROM's inherent ability to store large amounts of data and to provide rapid access times on inexpensive personal computers; second, the CD-ROM's ability to use large image, sound, and movie files. The popularity of the CD-ROM format is due not exclusively to these attractive qualities, but also to the current limitations of Internet technology. Commercially, the Internet currently does not contain a well-developed charging and reimbursement mechanism, making its use for publishing companies a second priority. Additionally, current Internet access occurs via regular phone dial-ups with 28.8K or 56K baud modems, and this translates into prohibitive teaching file transfer times. For example, an average case with four images and a half-page of text (at times up to 1.5 Mb of information) can take in excess of 15 minutes to transfer. With the advent of broadband connection methods to the Internet and newer compression algorithms, these problems are beginning to be resolved.

Despite these current limitations, there is great benefit in having the ability to adopt a server-client model in which central updates on the "server" are instantaneously reflected to all users or "clients." It is this aspect of teaching files on the WWW that is most appealing to educators. With value-added services offered along with these teaching files, including continuing medical education (CME) credit and advertising, this medium should prove very popular for practicing radiologists.

Commercially, as an electronic migration occurs of film-based teaching files, the future is on-line Internet-based teaching files. As publishers develop charging mechanisms and put CME credit into place, this method will become commonplace. Currently, due to limitations in these areas, most publishers are continuing to chose the CD-ROM format for its familiarity and traditional reimbursement mechanisms. For the personal users and educators, the Internet is available, ready, and capable of housing an electronic teaching file that the radiologic community can use.

Creating an Internet-Based Teaching File

Creating an Internet-based teaching file is a three-step process (Figure 4-1). First, the necessary images for case review must be obtained and, if not already in a native digital format, must be converted. This conversion process can be performed through various mechanisms, the most popular of which are discussed below. Second, the necessary teaching textual data must be added to the images and the case as a whole to convey the educator's teaching points. Third, the educator must have a means to organize all the elements of the teaching file with the various cases and textual data, a task that can be performed with a conventional Web page creation software package, such as Microsoft FrontPage and Adobe Sitemill. For users who wish to use public domain software, there are shareware versions available on the Internet that will allow the creation of the final electronic teaching case.

Step 1: Obtaining Digital Images

Converting Analog Film

If the images to be used in the teaching files are on film, one of two "analog to digital converting" devices can be used. The first is a film digitizer—a device

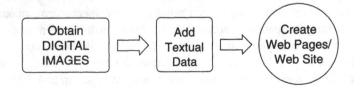

FIGURE 4.1. Stages in creating an electronic internet-based teaching file.

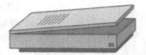

FIGURE 4.2. A typical film digitizer.

that uses a variety of technologies to create a digital replica of the analog film-based image (Figure 4-2). Essentially, a film is processed through this scanner, and a digital representation of the original film is produced. There are various technologies employed inside the scanners, including CCD and laser, to perform this conversion.

If your images are on slides, slide scanners are available that will convert the analog information on the slide negative to a digital format for use in electronic teaching files (Figure 4-3).

An alternate method, now becoming more common, is the use of a digital camera that performs a task similarly to the digitizer but is far more portable (Figure 4-4). Digital cameras come in many varieties and have many options. In general, for most radiologic applications, one should use a 2-megapixel or 2K × 2K camera to ensure a resolution that is adequate for subtle findings. The range of camera resolutions in the marketplace is 340 × 280 pixels or 4K × 4K cameras. The costs of the 4-megapixel cameras are currently prohibitive for home applications, but most 2K to 3K cameras fall into an affordable price range. While the 2K resolution is adequate for your teaching file needs, you may wish to have a higher resolution for home projects and family portrait albums. In general, the higher the resolution of the camera, the "crisper" the digital images acquired.

Once the film-based images have been converted from analog (film) format to a digital (scanner, slide scanner, or digital camera) format, the images can be manipulated on the computer. The most popular image editing software packages including Adobe Photoshop, Microsoft Paint, and Corel Draw; however,

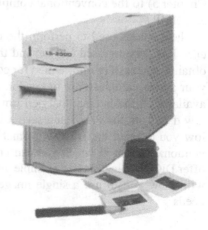

FIGURE 4.3. A typical slide digitizer. (Reproduced with permission from Nikon, Inc.)

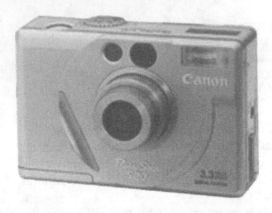

FIGURE 4.4. A typical digital camera. (Reproduced with permission from Canon America, Inc.)

shareware or public domain free versions of similar software packages are available on the Internet (visit *www.download.com*). With these image-editing software packages you will be able to crop, adjust, edit, and enhance the images to convey the teaching message that you desire. In addition, you are able to add textual data to the image and annotations in the form of arrows. After all your adjustments are made, you are able to save the images in a format previously discussed, including JPEG, TIFF, or BMP, and display them on the WWW/ Internet.

Transferring Already-Existing Digital Images

An alternate situation exists for many users when the images already are available in a digital format due to the use of a departmental picture archiving communication system (PACS) or Web distribution server. In this case, these images can be saved from these systems to the desktop and included in Web-based teaching files using the aforementioned tools. The harvest of images from the PACS usually involves the conversion of the DICOM format (see Chapter 5) to the conventional compression protocols, including JPEG, TIFF, and BMP.

The methods used to perform the conversion task are individual to the specific PACS being used and beyond the scope of this book. You can, however, obtain the necessary information for conversion and transmission of images from your system administrator or vendor. Alternatively, there are shareware utilities available on the Internet that perform DICOM conversion. After you obtain the raw data from the PACS and save it to your PC, these conversion tools will allow you to open the DICOM format images and convert them to a more conventional format in which you can perform editing tasks. Several vendors also offer DICOM plug-ins (for example, *www.desacc.com*) for Adobe Photoshop that will allow you to use a single image editing program for all your adjustment needs.

Step 2: Adding Textual Data

Adding textual data can be done in two ways. For the beginner, it usually is easiest to add image-related textual information right onto the image. By creating two versions of an image, one with the text and one without the text, the user can first view the "clean" image and then click on a button to move to the next Web page, where the image, with the annotation and textual data, is displayed. This provides a sequential learning experience and is relatively simple for the educator to create. The textual data and annotation as described above can be added in different popular image editing program, such as Adobe Photoshop, Microsoft Picture It, and Corel Draw, to name a few.

For the more advanced user, textual data can be created on Web pages that surround the image. For examples of this type of teaching file method, visit the teaching file sections on *www.auntminnie.com* or *www.radcom.org*. With this method, one needs a little more experience in Web page creation, but the finished product is quite impressive. What is comforting is that most Web page creation tools currently available offer a step-by-step approach that will guide you through the development of a website.

In general, the textual data are best added in separate elements; for example, the history of the case can be included on the first Web page (Figure 4-5). On this screen will help you to move through the other Web pages in the case. Next,

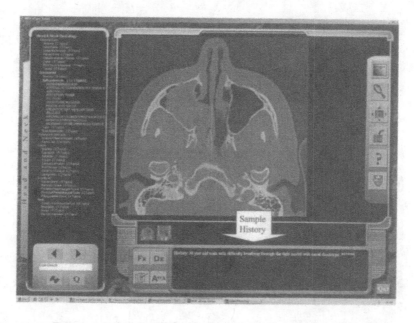

FIGURE 4.5. Sample Web page showing presentation of history.

the images of the case are presented in sequential order with any necessary information. At this point, the educator can make available the findings by displaying the images with the annotations that were previously created through the image editing program (Figure 4-6). Lastly, the diagnosis and discussion can be presented on the final Web page (Figure 4-7).

Step 3: Distribution

Once you have created all the elements of your teaching file case either in a Web page creation program or independently using HTML, the case needs to be placed on a Web server. There are three options that will make your teaching file material available on the WWW. First, many ISPs offer space on their servers when you purchase Internet access from them. Second, many users will upload their Web pages to this space and make the specific address to this Web page available to other users. Third, several of the popular Web page creation software tools offer "Web server" software within their packages. If you have a full-time Internet connection and can afford to have a Web server software package running in the background of your computer, this may be an option for you. Remember that there are issues regarding security if you host a Web server on your own home computer, and the novice user should beware! The last option, one users often prefer, is to upload the Web page information to a server in the radiology department. With this option, a member of the IS department of the hos-

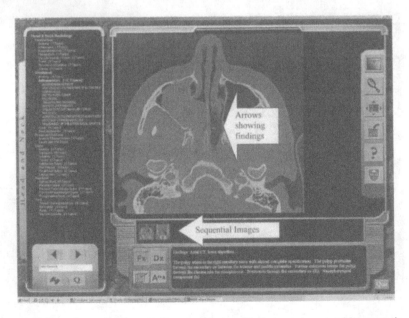

FIGURE 4.6. Sample follow-up Web page showing findings on image with annotation in the form of arrows.

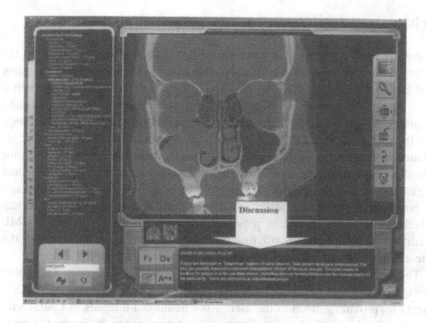

FIGURE 4.7. Sample Web page showing discussion following history and findings.

pital can worry about firewall issues. Often, the Web page address is linked to the institutional Web page, thus offering more publicity for your Web page.

Step 4: Viewing Your Teaching File

For users to view the Internet-based teaching file you have created, they can use any commonly available Web browser and receive information through their Internet connection. There often are locations where Internet access is not available on demand. In this situation, you can place the Web pages you have created on a CD-ROM that also contains the browser software and physically send this CD-ROM to the intended user. By installing the browser software, if not already available, a user can view the Web pages on the CD; you have created a virtual Internet connection except that you are acting not only as the client but also as the server in the local environment. The downside to this method is that the CD-ROMs need to be distributed physically.

In the recent past, some users have created software packages that are specific to radiology and to the creation of radiologic teaching files. These packages often streamline the creation of a case, since they offer the tools to input history, findings, and discussion as well as to annotate and edit images. Some of the more robust packages will allow export of the teaching file, once completed, in the form of HTML Web pages for uploading to a Web server or in the form of a self-contained teaching file for CD-ROM distribution.

What About CME?

There are many different commercial sites that offer teaching cases on the Internet. Several of these offer images and discussion, while others offer questions and CME credit. Many teaching files are used as material to attract users to a Web site so that they will use other services available there. If you are interested in providing CME for teaching files that are created on and distributed through the Internet, it is best to contact the CME department of your institution or affiliated university. In certain regions, hospitals are able to grant CME credit for grand rounds lectures and similar educational symposia; sometimes professional organizations also can grant CME credit; in other instances, only the university is granted that ability. The specifics of your institution most often will dictate whether you would be able to provide CME credit. For users to obtain CME credit on Web sites already offering on-line CME, they must register with the site and provide the necessary contact and payment information.

The arena of on-line CME is still in development. There are many issues that exist, including the governing body that grants the CME credit and the requirements for providing credit to the user. Since traditional methods of CME credit have revolved around educational instruction at meetings in the form of lectures and question-and-answer sessions, questions have been raised about the validity of this new method of learning. Nonetheless, there are several companies and institutions currently offering CME on the WWW in the form of lectures that stream over the Internet connection to your computer. By watching the lecture and answering a set of questions, a user can earn several hours of CME credit for which documentation is provided. As this new industry will still be evolving over the next several years, an in-depth discussion now would be premature. Keep an eye out for future developments. Maybe someday you will be sitting on the beach in Hawaii viewing CME streaming media on your laptop through a satellite connection!

Part III
Technologies Revolutionizing Radiology

5
PACS: Picture Archiving and Communication Systems

Image Acquisition
Image Archiving
  Short Term
    Random Access Memory
    Magnetic Disk
  Medical Short Term
    RAID (Redundant Array of Inexpensive
      Disks)
  Long Term

Compact Disk Recordable (CDR)
DVD (Digital Versatile Disk)
Optical Disk
DLT (Digital Linear Tape)
Image Transmission
Image Interpretation
ACR Standards
Conclusion

The advent of digital imaging has led to a revolution within the medical arena and has resulted in the development of picture archiving and communication systems (PACS). In common parlance, PACS means different things to different people. It is a unique technology in that it affects and applies to the practice of a broad range of individuals, including physicians (both radiologists and nonradiologists), technologists, administrators, vendors, and information technology (IT) professionals. To some radiologists, PACS often does not extend past the system that acquires, delivers, and stores the medical images interpreted each day. For others, it represents a great resource for research, education, and future developments. For referring physicians, it can mean easy remote access to the images of their patients as well as improved turnaround times and patient care. For technologists, it can mean streamlined operations, more time to perform examinations, and less time spent on filming and placing stickers. For administrators, it can mean not only saved monies and personnel and physical space, but also capital expenditure and cost justification strategies.

Prior to focusing in-depth on the PACS technology, there are key elements forming the infrastructure of a digital enterprise that need to be discussed. First, there is the Radiology Information System (RIS). The RIS is a subdivision of the Hospital Information System (HIS), the system that maintains the majority of electronic patient data. The RIS is responsible for all aspects of the work flow within a radiology department, from scheduling to billing to reporting. Second, there is the imaging network or the PACS. This technology encompasses elements such as workstations, archives, networks, and acquisition devices that enable the digital creation, transfer, and storage of medical data.

PACS encompasses a broad range of technologies that facilitate digital radiology. At the most fundamental level, PACS represents the integration of image acquisition devices, display workstation, and storage systems—all connected via a computer network. The early systems of the 1980s typically served single functions in order to solve single operational problems within a department. As the technology blossomed over the past two decades, more complicated and encompassing systems were developed, with current offerings allowing complete conversion to digital acquisition, transfer, interpretation, storage, and transmission.

The integration of the RIS, the HIS, and the PACS solves many of the issues of image generation, manipulation, interpretation, and dictation within the radiology department. However, the largest impetus behind this electronic migration is the elimination of film.

The delivery of radiologic services in many departments hinges on the use of radiographic film, now termed a legacy system. The work flow of imaging studies traditionally commences with a manually completed and scheduled request sent by a referring physician. Once the study has been scheduled into a queue, the patient is imaged, and film-based images are printed. This film subsequently is correlated with prior imaging studies the patient has had performed, and these are arranged for interpretation and dictation. Once the films are reviewed by a radiologist, a report is dictated and transcribed by a transcription service and ultimately sent to the referring physician. Several forms of distribution exist in various departments for provision of reports to the referring physician, from telephone and fax to a fully developed HIS.

Attempts are now in progress to automate each aspect of the imaging process, with the PACS automating the processes within the radiology department from image delivery to storage and billing. These processes are slowly being integrated as departments make the transition to fully digital enterprises. See Figure 5-1 for a diagram of a full departmental PACS.

Activity within the digital department begins with on-line order entry via distributed terminals or WWW-based entry protocols. Upon entry, the order is scheduled within the RIS. Concurrently, this information is passed on to a broker within the PACS to ensure timely retrieval of prior studies for comparison. Once the patient has been imaged, the acquired images become available to the enterprise. The distribution of images to the enterprise routinely is accomplished through various means including, but not limited to, the Internet.

A specific list of PACS vendors is not included here, since this list changes quite frequently. There are many resources available on the Internet (see Chapter 9) that provide links to vendors. In addition, vendors should be more than willing to provide information and contacts for other competitors so that you may compare problems.

Image Acquisition

Nearly 60% of the relative value unit (RVU) of imaging today comes from cross-sectional digital modalities. These modalities include computed tomography (CT), magnetic resonance imaging (MRI), and ultrasound. The remain-

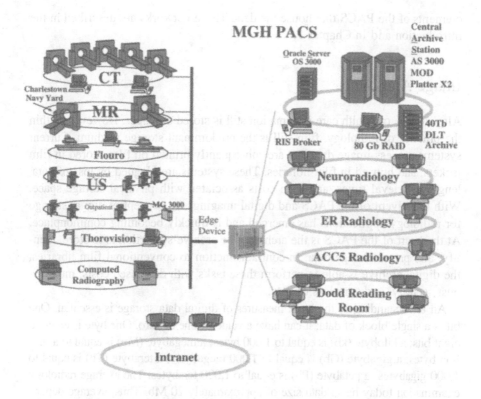

FIGURE 5.1. Sample diagram of a full departmental PACS.

ing imaging services include radiography, encompassing conventional to interventional radiographs and mammography. For true integration into the digital department, it is necessary for devices producing images to be capable of producing digital data in a conventional format. CT, MRI, and ultrasound acquisition devices produce digital output, with most current systems offering Digital Imaging and Communications in Medicine (DICOM) protocols for communication. Many older systems that were installed prior to definition of the DICOM standard often do not offer DICOM connectivity; in these cases, there are third-party add-on devices that perform conversion. Since a large portion of imaging volume is produced by radiography, the integration of plain film radiography into a digital architecture is paramount. Currently, radiographic devices are available in two formats: analog (often termed conventional) and digital (often referred to as computed radiography). The distinction between these imaging systems becomes important when determining whether the modality is capable of producing the necessary digital data for integration into the digital department. Emerging onto the marketplace are mammographic devices that produce digital output, but currently their costs are significantly higher than those of their analog counterparts. Once acquired, these image data are then transmitted over the network to the workstations, archives, and other elements of the PACS that house the data. These networks are described in the introduction and in Chapter 1.

Image Archiving

Almost 90% of health care information still is stored on paper. However, within the practice of radiology, film still is the predominant storage medium. Current systems process image data that are subsequently printed on film, stored in film jackets, and housed in film libraries. These systems are plagued by loss of data, lengthy retrieval times, and high costs associated with physical storage space. With the advent of the PACS and digital imaging, the concept of digital storage for radiology applications has emerged and is quickly becoming commonplace. At the heart of the PACS is the archive. The archive's function is to store, identify, and protect image data. In contradistinction to conventional film libraries, the digital archive is able to perform these tasks with decreased costs, more robust security, and zero loss of data.

An understanding of the basic measures of digital data storage is essential. One bit is a single block of data; it can have a value of one or zero. One byte is equal to eight bits; a kilobyte (kb) is equal to 1,000 bytes; a megabyte (Mb) is equal to a million bytes; a gigabyte (Gb) is equal to 1,000 megabytes; a terabyte (Tb) is equal to 1,000 gigabytes; a petabyte (Pb) is equal to 1,000 terabytes. The average radiology examination today has a data size of approximately 20 Mb. Thus, average departments performing 100,000 imaging studies per year require 10 to 20 Gb of local on-line storage, usually hundreds of gigabytes of near-line storage, and 2 to 4 Tb of long-term storage. There are various archiving levels required in a filmless environment, from immediate access memory to near-line storage to deep archive storage. The options for solutions at each of these archiving levels are described below.

Short Term

Random Access Memory

Random access memory (RAM) found in the desktop PC is a data storage medium. The speed to access data from RAM is not affected by the order in which it is stored on the hardware. The most common form of RAM in use today is built from semiconductor integrated circuits. RAM can be configured in sizes of up to 1 Gb, and access to data can occur in the nanosecond range.

Magnetic Disk

A hard drive in a desktop PC is a flat rotating disk covered on one or both sides with magnetizable material. To store information, small areas or "zones" on a magnetic disk are magnetized. Data are read and written by a head that is positioned at various parts of the disk by a spinning mechanism. Hard disks have an access time of 20 to 30 msec and can store up to 20 Gb of data.

Medium Short Term

RAID (Redundant Array of Inexpensive Disks)

A redundant array of inexpensive disks (RAID) consists of hard disk drives linked together in series. RAIDs increase data protection and availability, increase total storage capacity, and provide performance flexibility. Performance can be increased by spreading data and performing operations in parallel, allowing multiple drivers to be working on a single input or output request. RAID configurations can store up to 1 Tb of data and have access times similar to those of magnetic spinning disks or hard drives.

Long Term

Compact Disk Recordable (CDR)

Compact disk recordable (CDR) is a user recordable compact disk, a format that is routinely available both in the retail industry and now at home. CDR technology creates a CD-ROM disk that provides 650 Mb of storage per disk. CD-ROM jukeboxes and library systems provide fast, high-volume, permanent storage capabilities. Conventional CD-ROM jukeboxes can house from 200 Gb to 1 Tb of data, depending on the number of platters and disk changers, with average access times for random queries (incorporating the robotic arm change time) in the range of seconds.

DVD (Digital Versatile Disk)

Digital Versatile Disk (DVD) is a relatively new format in the storage industry. DVD physically comes in two formats: a two-layer single- or double-sided disk with capacities of 8.5 or 17 Gb, or a single-layer single- or double-sided disk with capacities of 4.7 or 9.4 Gb. DVD drives are backward compatible with the current CD-ROM format, so single DVD drives can meet both requirements. Average access times are similar to those of the CDR format.

Optical Disk

Magneto optical disks are $5^{1}/_{4}$ inches in diameter and are coated with a material that has special properties. Optical disks come in two varieties—write once read many (WORM) and magneto optical (MO)—with the MO disks being rewriteable many times. Conventionally, optical disks can hold up to 2.6 Gb of data, and when they are linked into a jukebox with a conventional number of platters, they can hold 1.3 Tb of data.

DLT (Digital Linear Tape)

Digital linear type (DLT) employs magnetic tape drives as a storage medium. DLT drives use a tape cartridge that is 4.1 inches square and 1 inch high and holds a $^1/_2$-inch metal-particle magnetic tape. DLTs are $^1/_2$-inch wide, and the cartridges come in several capacities, ranging from 20 to over 40 Gb.

Image Transmission

The ultimate benefit of digital data is the ability to transport them to multiple locations in real time concurrently. The transport of data through a radiology department and the entire enterprise allows almost simultaneous availability of images to all points connected to the network. The advent of the production of digital (usually DICOM) data has simplified drastically the processing and transmission of data by defining standard protocols and routines that each device can comprehend. This convention is utilized for routine tasks, including digital transmission, production of film for subsequent hard-copy interpretation, and storage in a central archive.

The advantages of specific network technologies, such as T1, T3, integrated services digital network (ISDN), and asynchronous digital subscriber line (ADSL), are varied. There are nuances in the technologies that result in different levels of performance. However, the common factor remains that each of the listed technologies is capable of using the Transmission Control Protocol/Internet Protocol (TCP/IP). This protocol is the standard communications protocol used throughout the Internet, thereby ensuring stability and vendor support. The use of these protocol technologies also permits the department or hospital local area network to extend to remote sites by means of a side-area network.

Image Interpretation

Once data enter a central location or computer system within a digital department, the images can be routed to various points within the network for purposes such as storage, interpretation, matching with prior examinations, logging/validation procedures, and eventual matching with the interpretation for reporting and billing purposes. In a fully integrated enterprise, these features are inherent to the PACS.

A key function in the work flow and in the role of a radiologist is primary interpretation of images. This task in this new environment is performed on workstations that are directly connected to the central PACS and indirectly connected to remote imaging centers via the Internet or the Intranet. These workstations deliver images to the radiologist from any location for interpretation in another location. The typical scenario encompasses the integration of information from the RIS as an aid to the reporting radiologist. The final link is through the HIS to the enterprise. The current workstation configurations that are commercially available commonly utilize the Unix operating system and custom-designed software. Usually, the software running on these high-end workstations is geared toward image interpretation and manipulation, with multiple tools available for image manipulation, including window and level, brightness, contrast, markup, annotation, and measure. Most iterations of workstation software allow radiologists to create worklists, based on indicators of study status (from new to reported), that ultimately allow efficient monitoring of work flow during a workday.

ACR Standards

As the PACS is integrated into our daily radiology practice more and more, it is important to be sure that the highest levels of quality and management standards are maintained. The American College of Radiology (ACR) publishes standards on the practice of radiology. Any discussion of PACS should include the issues and specifications addressed in the ACR document entitled "ACR Standard for Digital Image Data Management." For your benefit, we have reproduced this document in its entirety in Appendix 1 at the end of this book.

Conclusion

From discussions with leaders in the radiology community, it is evident that the Internet, digital imaging, and specifically PACS are creating a revolution, and that most departments eventually will perform digital radiology in one form or another. In this decade, hundreds of hospitals will convert to PACS and enterprise-level imaging. Due to the numerous benefits, the adoption of this technology is inevitable, and a keen understanding of the key components can be useful to every aspect of daily practice.

6
Teleradiology

Teleradiology has been the subject of entire textbooks. The topic is of paramount importance to radiologists and radiology personnel. This chapter provides an overview of the technology and the impact the Internet has had in its growth and development, familiarizing you with the issues that exist and, it is hoped, sparking your interest to explore this area further for your own practice. For the specifics regarding financial, legal, and administrative issues in setting up and maintaining a teleradiology practice, other resources and references are available. Vendors that provide teleradiology services have not been included here since this list evolves and changes on a daily basis. There are many resources on the Internet that provide links to vendors (see Chapter 9).

History and Perspective

Teleradiology is one of the most developed forms of telemedicine. It can be defined as the delivery of health care and the sharing of medical expertise using a telecommunications system. Telemedicine does not define the distance over which medical information is shared, although the recipients of care are typically thought to be outside the local area of the caregivers. From a purely historical perspective, the telephone remains the standard method for communicating medical information. Teleradiology itself became an entity in the 1960s when Kenneth T. Bird, M.D., of the Massachusetts General Hospital (MGH) used an interactive television and a direct microwave link to connect Logan Airport in Boston and MGH, approximately 3 miles away.

The feasibility of telemedicine was first recognized in a program sponsored by the government, the Space Technology Applied to Rural Papago Advanced Health Care (STARPAHC) program. This project, funded by the National Aeronautics and Space Administration (NASA), sought to utilize monitoring systems developed for use in space to serve the Papago Reservation. While the program proved the feasibility of telemedicine in a rural setting, it was not cost-effective or practical. The Department of Defense and its initiatives in developing telemedicine technologies for the battlefield have had a huge impact on the development of these technologies for the civilian sector.

Since the 1960s, the fields of telemedicine and teleradiology showed little advance outside military applications. It was not until the early 1990s that realistic bandwidths became available for the transmission of large data files. As bandwidth and compression algorithms became more commonplace by the mid-1990s, implementation of teleradiology increased dramatically in the United States. In addition, the development of radiologic modalities and adjunct devices that could either send or capture images and other data in a digital, electronic form helped popularize the technology. With the development of interactive video conferencing systems for the business world, telemedicine and teleradiology began to become realities.

Digitizing Images

To transmit a radiologic image over telecommunications systems, the image must be converted into a digital format. Many modalities produce images that are inherently digital, including CT, MRI, ultrasound, nuclear medicine, computer radiography (CR), and digital radiography (DR). If an image is produced on hardcopy film, it, too, can be transmitted once digitized.

Image formats that comply with the Digital Image Communication in Medicine standard provide predictable results. A DICOM-3–compliant system will produce digital images from an acquisition device without loss of the full 12-bit data set (2,056 gray scale). It ensures no image degradation and the full capability of the radiologist receiving the image to adjust the image window and level settings through their full complement. Since much of the older equipment that is currently used in teleradiology is not DICOM compliant, alternate solutions have been sought.

The most common method used to perform this task has been the scanner solution. A digital rendition is created from a copy of the film by digitizing the image with a laser or by using a CCD digitizer. Older solutions include the use of a video frame grabber, which converts the video signal output of a modality, such as the CT console, to a digital form, producing an image.

File Sizes

There are several factors that require balancing for teleradiology to become an effective technology. Typically, the file sizes for digital images are very large, ranging from hundreds of kilobytes to 40 to 50 megabytes. It can take many hours to transmit these large files across standard phone lines. The complicating factors for teleradiology practices are twofold: the increasing number of studies performed on patients when they are evaluated for a single disease; and the new modalities, such as multislice CT, that can generate over 1,000 images per study. These factors have generated a large increase in the volume of information that needs to be transmitted. Although a single image from a CT study may not take very long to send from one site to another, a single slice is of limited utility to the radiologist interpreting the patient's studies. Hence, using conventional network transmission methods becomes expensive and impractical. Fortunately, the 1990s witnessed a revolution in the use of information technology, with rapidly increasing availability of bandwidth and the amount of information that could be sent per unit time. While this great increase helped ease the problem, it still often was impractical to perform teleradiology adequately. Thus, solutions were sought to make the image files smaller, yet retain all the radiologically relevant data.

Image Compression

Chapter 1 discusses image compression and the method by which a large file is reduced to a smaller file with or without loss of data. Teleradiology almost exclusively has used either the JPEG or wavelet forms of compression, which have proved to be both practical and powerful. Both these formats can be used in either a lossy or lossless mode and can be manipulated by the radiologist. The JPEG standard currently is the only format that is supported by the DICOM standard, but, with revisions of the standard, newer compression algorithms most likely will be explored.

Inherent in the JPEG format is the problem that images suffer from "block artifacts." These are artificial edges that are created between pixel blocks, especially at high compression ratios. Wavelet compression does not always suffer from the same problems, especially at higher compression ratios, and thus is often used in implementations of a teleradiology system. A major benefit of wavelet compression as compared with the JPEG format is that it will allow more flexibility with higher compression ratios while maintaining the image quality for interpretation. The compression ratio is directly related to the effective transfer rate of images over data lines, especially if teleradiology is employed as a real-time service.

Image Transmission

There currently are several types of data lines that can be utilized in implementing a teleradiology system. Several of these options are discussed in detail in Chapter 2. To reiterate here, these include the conventional dial-up telephone, broadband services such as cable modem, and DSL, ISDN, T1, T3, and ATM. Many small-volume teleradiology practices can use the ISDN or T1 solutions and provide excellent service. Compression ratios of at least 8–10:1 must be used to achieve manageable file sizes. The choice of which data line to use will vary with the type of teleradiology practice; for example, on call services may be able to use conventional dial-up telephone lines without any issues with transmission times of image/studies.

Image Interpretation

The interpretation of an image received from a teleradiology system usually is done on a workstation as a part of a PACS or on a home computer by an on-call radiologist. If a teleradiology system is integrated into a PACS, the image information can be sent over the LAN to multiple workstations or can be based on a subspecialty service. These images then can be archived or stored for the necessary time as outlined in the teleradiology agreement. Often, there is no archival requirement, since the images are stored by the sending institution or group. The type of monitor used to review studies depends primarily on the type of teleradiology system. For conventional "on-call" services, lower resolutions adequately provided by home computers can be utilized. The American College of Radiology (ACR) has made recommendations as to minimum standards for primary interpretation.

Report Generation

It is the generated report that is of paramount importance to the referring clinician or to the radiologist sending images via a teleradiology system. The Internet has provided many new ways to send reports produced by conventional dictation systems; these include e-mail, fax, and text-to-speech over the phone. If a voice recognition system is integrated into a teleradiology system, many of the manual functions can be automated; the radiologist's report, once validated, can automatically be sent via one of these methods, as authentication is instantaneous once the radiologist signs the report. This often can save hours on report generation times.

Security

Any discussion of transmission of patient data over the Internet must include the issues of security and confidentiality of patient data. Michael M. Medenis of the University of Arizona discusses in-depth many of the issues and requirements regarding security in teleradiology at *www.ece.arizona.edu/~medenis/hw2/sem_pro.htm*.

Many of the governing factors surrounding transmission of data in teleradiology and telemedicine are addressed in the Health Information Portability Accountability Act (HIPAA) of 1996, which was enacted as part of a broad congressional attempt at incremental health care reform. The goal of this act was to develop standards and requirements for maintenance and transmission of health information that identifies individual patients. In general, these standards were designed for two reasons: first, to improve the efficiency and effectiveness of the health care system by standardizing the interchange of electronic data for specified administrative and financial transactions; and second, to protect the security and confidentiality of electronic health information.

A brief overview of the standards highlights four key areas: (1) information security, (2) privacy, (3) electronic data interchange, and (4) unique identifiers. The specific implementation of HIPAA in terms of teleradiology at the time of the publication of this book is not finalized. The bottom line, though, is that, once the final guidelines are published, all teleradiology practices will be required to HIPAA compliant in terms of the security measures or they will incur hefty fines. Currently, it is proposed that when the new HIPAA privacy standards take effect, they will mandate penalties for violating confidentiality provisions as follows: $100 per patient; $250,000 for willful misuse of private information. Because the standards are not set, many companies are enforcing security policies that are thought to be above and beyond the standards that will be set forth.

Current up-to-date information on the HIPAA standards can be obtained at the Department of Health and Human Services (DHHS) Web page at *http://aspe.hhs. gov/admnsimp/Index.htm.*

ACR Standards

As teleradiology develops, it is important to be sure that certain levels of quality are maintained. The American College of Radiology (ACR) publishes standards on the practice of radiology. Any discussion of teleradiology should include the issues and specifications addressed in the ACR document entitled "ACR Standard for Teleradiology." For your benefit, we have reproduced this document in its entirety in Appendix 2 at the end of this book.

Conclusion

For teleradiology to be cost-effective, some method is required to reduce the file sizes of digitized images without compromising image quality. Compression algorithms are the solution to this problem, especially for large medical image files. These algorithms can compress images down to 20 to 30 times their original size and can make transmission fast and inexpensive. This transmission occurs over a myriad of options, from phone lines to dedicated data cable lines. Once received at the interpretation site, the images can be decompressed and either sent to dedicated workstations or home computers or integrated into a LAN or a PACS for interpretation. Once the report is completed, it can be sent back to the referring physician via the Internet using e-mail, fax, or phone. This process often can be improved with the use of voice recognition technology.

The current state of technology allows teleradiology to be a feasible addition to the radiology practice. It helps radiology serve both underserviced areas as well as locations where subspecialty consultative services are not readily available. In the future, the impact of teleradiology most likely will continue to be felt in three areas. First, teleradiology's ability to provide subspecialty consultation to areas that do not possess these skills will supplement a growing user base. With the shortage of manpower growing in radiology, the ability to centralize subspecialty services by using a teleradiology infrastructure will enable general radiologists to continue to provide the bulk of services to the population. Second, teleradiology will allow interactive examinations, such as ultrasound, to be performed in remote health centers while under the supervision of a radiologist. Third, teleradiology will allow provision of expert radiologic consultation in the emergency setting on a 24-hour basis. Most likely, this initially will be on an on-call consultative basis, but, once volume reaches a point where it is constant, especially in heavy-volume practices, utilizing time zone differences in various parts of the country or world will allow night coverage during day hours at varied geographic locations.

7
Voice Recognition

There are many new technologies being developed that are revolutionizing the practice of radiology. Dictation is an integral part of our day-to-day practice and represents an area in which improvements would save us both time and money. Advances in speech and voice recognition (VR) technology have brought about more practical, usable speech recognition capabilities in the past five years. In late 1994, the effort to develop large-vocabulary, continuous speech recognition systems in American English had progressed to the point where accuracy had become less of an issue and vendors could focus on specific markets. In addition, the development of the Internet and intranets created an infrastructure with a client-server model that could support such a dictation system.

In a recent informal worldwide membership survey, the Healthcare Information Management and Systems Society found that 31% of respondents were eager to install VR systems in their practices. No specialty was more eager or better suited than radiology. To date, radiologists have handled the process of dictation either by manually writing the report or by recording the report on tape and then having it processed by medical transcriptionists. This mode of dictation and transcription is both time-consuming and expensive.

The choice of transcribing radiology reports with voice recognition systems is feasible due to the consistent and predictable vocabulary within most dictation practices. This chapter will give you a basic understanding of both the technology and the issues you will face when discussing your implementation with a potential vendor.

Technology

VR software encompasses, at the highest level, four core processes or technologies: spoken recognition of human speech, synthesis of human readable characters into speech, speaker identification and verification, and comprehension.

These are referred to as speech recognition (or speech-to-text), speech synthesis (or text-to-speech), speaker identification and verification, and natural language understanding (NLU).

Speech Recognition

Speech recognition is the technology that makes it possible for the computer to translate the spoken word into type. There are two distinct types of speech we use in our day-to-day lives. The first type is command and the second type is continuous. Thus, there are two types of voice recognition: the first type is termed spoken command recognition, also known as command and control, and the second type is termed continuous dictation. Command and control dictation handles the recognition of single words or short phrases spoken with continuous speech, such as "Begin Dictation" or "Accept and Sign." This discrete dictation technology is easier for computers to handle, since it has lower processing power requirements; however, it cannot be used in routine dictation, since it requires the user to place a short pause between each spoken word. Continuous dictation, as the term implies, does not carry this limitation and thus is employed in the radiology context.

Speech Synthesis

Speech synthesis, also referred to as text-to-speech, is the technology that makes it possible for the computer to produce the phonemes we make when we read text out loud. Within radiology, speech synthesis allows the radiologist to listen to a review of the entire report once he has finished dictating it as well as to playback portions just dictated.

Speaker Identification and Verification

Speaker identification and verification are two related technologies. These technologies, unlike speech recognition and speech synthesis, deal with the identity of the human speaker and not with what was spoken or with synthesizing the particular human voice. With speaker verification, technology is applied to authenticate a given human speaker against a database pool of enrolled candidates. The advantage this technology affords the user is that the computer can store specific nuances in the individual's voice that can help improve dictation accuracies. This can be of paramount importance in practices in which there may be users of various regional backgrounds with different accents.

Natural Language Understanding

Natural language understanding (NLU) is the technology that makes it possible for the computer to understand the meaning of either the words dictated or the text typed. Hence, NLU will allow the computer to understand a query or statement put forth by the radiologist in natural human language. This means understanding not simply the words spoken, but the meaning behind them. Although this sounds like a useful technology, the applications in pure dictation are limited. However, when integrated into a complete system, this will allow the radiologist, for example, to simply ask the computer to "show all new CTs that have not been dictated between eight o'clock last night and now; the system, in turn, will then generate the appropriate list.

Software

There are many vendors currently on the market that are offering voice recognition packages for the public. Most radiology packages contain a 25,000 radiology-oriented vocabulary and average advertised accuracy rates of over 95% for most American English speakers. Although vendors boast that no special training in the software is required, most radiologists have found that their recognition accuracy benefits from completing a short enrollment in the system during which individual voice nuances are detected and stored for future analysis. The language model used in the system allows it to distinguish between words and symbols that sound alike, such as "to," "two," and "too," or the symbol for the punctuation mark "colon" and a patient's anatomic colon. Macros can be created to generate sections of a radiology report with a single word. There are key features of VR software that you, as a potential user, should be sure are available within any package you consider for deployment in your practice. These features are discussed below.

Open RIS/HIS Interface

Any VR package should contain an interface to download demographic data directly to the VR package and upload the finalized radiology reports to be stored directly onto the RIS/HIS. To achieve this link, the software must contain a documented Hospital Language 7 (HL-7)-compliant application programming interface, with standard format and standard protocols. A more detailed understanding of this portion of the software is not required for successful deployment.

Prestored Reports

The individual radiologist or institution should be able to create sets of canned text reports (a "normal chest," for example) and store them with a single command word or acronym for later recall. When displayed, the prestored report can be further customized or simply signed as a final report.

Templates

A radiologist should be able to create standardized report format templates that will make dictation faster for procedure-based subspecialties. The template capability gives the radiologist the ability to create a form with fill-in-the-blank areas and recall them with a simple macro command. The radiologist then dictates the words needed to fill in the blanks. This feature also allows institutions to capture key data elements, such as medication dosing, catheter sizes, or contrast doses.

Addendum

This feature gives the radiologist the capability to add additional information to a final or signed report while maintaining the integrity of the existing report. This information can be shared with other information systems, such as a radiology or hospital system, through the RIS interface agent.

User-Defined Fields

There should be a number of user-defined fields that give an institution the flexibility to input additional information, such ICD9 codes, CPT codes, ACR/NEMA codes, or any other information an institution deems necessary to collect at the time a report is created. This information can be shared with other information systems, such as a radiology or hospital system, through the RIS interface agent.

Bar Code Interface

A standard VR package should include a standard bar code interface that users can modify to suite their own bar code environment. This allows practices that generate tracking forms with bar codes to simply swipe the bar code instead of typing or entering the accession number for the study each time.

System Security

A user ID and password protection at sign-on and password reentry should be available so that the system can employ electronic signature of reports and ensure the security of patient information.

VR: One Story

Understanding the experiences of others always will help you in successfully deploying new systems in your own practice. While the installation of a VR system in many aspects is specific to your location, our experience will help clarify some of the steps along the way. The Massachusetts General Hospital conducts over 500,000 imaging studies per year. The annual transcription operating cost per annum was estimated to be nearly $1.2 million. The average turnaround time for a report to reach the referring physician during the transcription era had been 4.1 days. With such lengthy report times, the radiology department suffered delayed result reporting as well as delayed billing. When reviewing the problems associated with the conventional transcription paradigm, several operational qualities were exposed. With conventional transcription systems, an inherent bottleneck existed from "bursty" dictation traffic: we were reporting a large number of our cases in the morning and the mid- to late afternoon. This becomes a moot issue with voice dictation. There was also an inherent delay in final report signing due to transcription delays. These issues led to high and variable operating costs that also were incompatible with our efforts to implement an electronic medical record system.

Implementation

Our experience with VR technology began in November 1995 when we became an alpha test site for the IBM MedSpeak/Radiology development effort. In conjunction with IBM (White Plains, NY), a beta version of this program was piloted within our teleradiology practice by January 1996, and, by September 1996, we had gone live with a first product release in one area of the department. With a positive initial experience, we felt we were ready to embark on a wider implementation. In October 1996, the musculoskeletal division was converted to complete VR deployment with a department-wide multiphase rollout that began in January 1997 and was completed in early 1999. Over 1,000 reports per day were produced.

Challenges and Improvements

With any initial adoption of VR technology, there will be issues regarding acceptance as well as issues with the technology.

We faced many obstacles in the deployment of VR that centered primarily around the user. It always is difficult to convince users to implement a technology into their practice when its utilization does not benefit them immediately. Some of the difficulty may have come from the fact that it always took longer to generate reports with earlier versions of VR than with the conventional dictation system, due to training, experience, and antiquated hardware. It also was difficult to provide incentives, since cost savings produced with VR systems (cutting transcription time) are achieved at the expense of the radiologist's time. As the technology improves and the process becomes more streamlined, this time will shrink more and more. As with any technology, there always is a learning curve. We have overcome many of these obstacles by ensuring that as much effort as possible has been made to manage the project and provide technical support, especially user-friendly and convenient training sessions. Much of our success has been achieved by stressing the benefits and by the removal of alternative dictation systems.

We will continue to see improvements in sound cards and microphones that will translate into improvements in recognition accuracy and software stability. The microphone probably is the single most critical hardware element in the total speech recognition solution. A microphone that provides noise-cancellation technology, either active or passive, becomes mandatory, especially in high traffic areas. Currently, we have experienced our most successful recognition with a Sennheiser microphone; however, the integrated Philips Speechmike (Philips Electronics, New York, NY) microphone, including bar code, trackball, and dictation functions, is ergonomically most appealing.

Benefits

Clearly, the predominant benefit of VR is decreased report turnaround times. Several studies have shown a tenfold decrease in report times, from completion of the study to finalization of the report. These reductions are bolstered by the inherent benefits through PACS. VR also serves to reduce costs; our initial budgets demonstrated a $350,000 savings in the first two years after completing only phase one of a three-phase implementation. Theoretically VR also serves to increase report accuracy, since radiologists finalize reports immediately after dictation without a transcription delay.

Conclusion

From our department's ten-year experience of exploring a variety of VR systems, we have concluded that VR is a technology that is finally ready for prime time use. VR benefits the radiology department as well as the health care enterprise. The benefits of implementation are significant, as are the challenges. With a strong business plan and implementation proposal, VR can be rolled out in an efficient manner that is both technically and financially sound. As radiology continues to acquire a larger percentage of the shrinking health care dollar, improved report turnaround times and decreased operating costs will become a necessity. Implementation of VR technology will help to position radiology departments for the challenging future ahead.

8
Electronic Medical Record and Patient Care Specific to Radiology

What Are the Benefits of the Electronic Patient
    Record?
  Standards
  Integration
  Telemedicine/Teleradiology and the EMR
The Internet and the EPR
  Internet-Based Medical Image Distribution
  Costs

EMR: One Story
  Getting to a Web-Based Solution
  Image Data Repository
  Caveats
  Hardware
  Image Flow/Work Flow
  Future Applications

Traditionally, the majority of patient data has been housed on paper. With the advent of the personal computer, many institutions have moved toward electronic versions of portions of this record. Most physicians, at some point in their practice, have used computer-based laboratory and pathology reporting systems. Although the computerization of the radiology record makes sense, the task is enormous and faces difficulties in communication and integration.

The computerization of the medical record has moved rapidly in the past few years. In many centers, all of the essential medical history, such as clinic visits, hospital admission notes, problem lists, allergies, orders, diagnostic tests, and medications, are kept in electronic form. When a physician sees a patient, the most pertinent information is instantly available on a computer in a usable form. Many health care providers also have started to enter patient information into the electronic medical record (EMR) application and to perform all patient management functions in an electronic form.

Understanding the scope of this subject requires knowing the definitions of the specific associated terms. These are listed in Table 8-1 and discussed throughout this chapter.

Next, an understanding of the various computer systems involved and the work flow of information within a health care enterprise is required. Figure 8-1 charts these systems and the work flow. Information is housed in various archives. While the terms are generic, the concept is expressed in their descriptor. Patient demographic information is housed in a "master patient index." This information covers all contact and historical information and is the key to indexing patients within the health care system. The usual indexing method employed is a medical record number (MRN). Linked by the MRN is further information regarding the patient's care, specifically, clinical information housed in a "clinical data repository" and radiology studies housed in an "image data repository." These repositories are simply large-scale archives that store information. The integra-

TABLE 8.1.

Electronic medical record (EMR): The portion of the patient encounter not captured by conventional information systems, typically ambulatory data, including chief complaint, progress notes, medications, allergies, history and physical examination (H&P), etc. Commonly referred to as the EMR. This term often is used to connote the entire set of electronic medical data on a patient.

Electronic patient record (EPR): The combination of conventional medical information systems data (lab; radiology; admissions, discharge, and transfer; etc.) and the (ambulatory) electronic medical record.

Longitudinal medical record (LMR): See Electronic patient record.

Electronic health record (EHR): The combination of the electronic patient record with data entered by the patient, including symptoms, reactions to treatments, and other historical events.

Medical content trusted authority: Internet publishers of medical data that have been deemed trusted for patient use. The method for validation of these sources is currently poorly defined.

Clinical data repository (CDR): A database of information gathered by querying the various medical information systems of a provider for the common presentation of electronic medical results.

Image data repository (IDR): A database of information gathered by querying the various medical imaging systems of a provider for the common presentation of medical image data.

Interface engine: A device used to allow the communication of disparate medical information systems, typically within one provider. Such a system is necessary for the common delivery of electronic order entry and results reporting of heterogeneous information systems.

Medical record number (MRN): A unique number used to identify and track a patient throughout a single provider.

Accession number: The number used to identify and track a specific test, procedure, or examination of a patient. While the accession number alone may not be unique, the combination of MRN and accession number should be unique within a single provider.

Master patient index (MPI): When two or more hospitals share patients, there is a need to find a common and unique numbering system for these individuals. Since each patient will have a different MRN at each hospital, a new numbering system must be created with links back to each hospital's MRN data. This new overarching medical record number (and the computer system that generates it) is commonly referred to as the master patient index.

Departmental information systems: The information systems used to schedule, track, order, report, and bill for procedures within various departments of the hospital. The RIS, or radiology information system, is an example.

Electronic order entry: The entering of medical orders through the use of a computer. A doctor, nurse, or other designate typically performs the entry.

Electronic result reporting: The display of medical test results through the use of a computer as opposed to paper or film.

ADT: Abbreviation for admit, transfer, and discharge (the data typically contained by the hospital information system, HIS).

tion and utilization of this information is performed via the information systems termed the "hospital information systems": in the case of laboratory data, for example, for subspecialty departments such as pathology or endoscopy, the "departmental information systems" perform this function; the picture archiving and communication system (PACS) performs this function for radiology. The collection of this information is stored, catalogued and organized through the synergism of these systems. For a physician reviewing this information, an electronic patient record (EPR) viewer and the EMR will synthesize this information and make it available in a clinically useful manner. With the help of secure con-

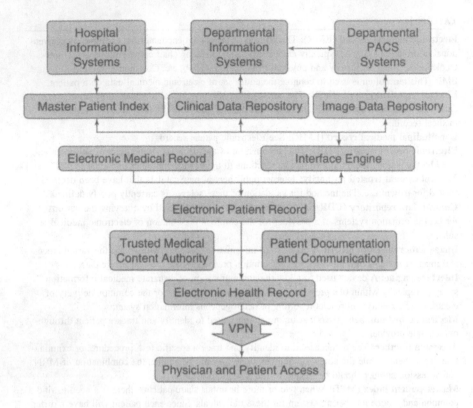

FIGURE 8.1. Medical patient information flow.

nections via virtual private networks (VPNs), this information can be made available to remote physicians and patients.

What Are the Benefits of the Electronic Patient Record?

Standards

The electronic medical record ensures a common structure for the patient record. With a common structure, there can be intercommunication between physicians and facilities of disparate locations and cultures. All of the incoming data, whether it is in the form of laboratory results or radiology images, follows the standard predefined format. See Figure 8-2 for the components of an electronic patient record. This ultimately means that the health care provider can devote a smaller amount of time to deciphering findings and a greater amount of time with the patient.

Integration

The paper-based electronic patient record allows sequential review of the patient data, usually in the form of one sheet of paper to the next. The use of computer-

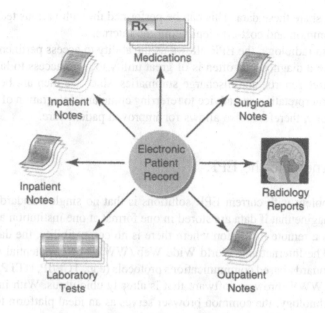

FIGURE 8.2. Components of the electronic patient record.

based EPR systems allows the physician to integrate potentially disparate, but relevant, data into all portions of the medical record, and to integrate and synthesize this information over time. For example, recent EKG results demonstrating atrial fibrillation may be relevant for both of the chief complaints of palpitations (cardiology) and left-sided weakness (neurology). Now, with the EPR, these data can be accessed simultaneously by both departments. In addition, a computer-based system allows the physician to study trends and patterns over time. For example, the physician easily can review the results of multiple chest x-rays obtained over the course of months to years when deciding if a nodule has grown. With patients suffering from specific disease processes that require careful charting or monitoring of lab values, including anticoagulation or blood sugar values, a computer-based system can provide other ways to present the data, including charts and graphs that can make it easier for patients to understand what is expected in their care.

Telemedicine/Teleradiology and the EMR

Another distinct benefit of the EPR is the ability to share patient data with remote locations. We have discussed the specifics of teleradiology in Chapter 6. The incorporation of all patient data into an electronic form allows physicians to offer many of the same benefits to their patients that teleradiology allows radiologists to offer to their patients. It is of increasing utility for physicians to be able to review prior routine lab tests and radiologic procedures performed by an outside institution or laboratory to save time and money in caring for a patient. Utilizing an electronic patient record allows physicians in different geographic locations to share these data. This can be performed through various techniques, the most common and cost-efficient being the Internet.

Specific to radiology, the EPR allows us the ability to access pertinent patient data to make a diagnosis. It often is of great utility to have access to laboratory data, operative reports, and discharge summaries, since we then are better able to provide interpretation and advice to referring clinicians. Integration of the EPR with radiology, therefore, also allows for improved patient care.

The Internet and the EPR

A large problem with current EPR solutions is that no single standard applies. One can imagine that if data are stored in one format at one institution and made available to a remote institution where there is no compatibility, the data are of no utility. The Internet and World Wide Web (WWW) offer potential solutions through standards-based communications protocols (e.g., TCP/IP, HTTP, and ActiveX) and WWW browser software that is already ubiquitous. With improving security technology, the common browser serves as an ideal platform to deliver medical data to the enterprise and beyond.

The challenge of incorporating radiologic images into the EPR is great. Many have proposed solutions to this problem, both in the commercial and academic markets. However, what unifies all of these solutions is the necessity to adhere to the conformity of standards for the transmission of both textual (HL-7) and image (DICOM) data. It ultimately is the integration of these two data sets that is clinically essential. The successful integration of radiologic image data as an adjunct to the textual data contained within the patient's electronic record thus can be achieved through the use of standard Internet protocols. The benefits of this integration are obvious. The remainder of this chapter addresses the problem of achieving this integration.

Internet-Based Medical Image Distribution

The legacy system of printed film allowed referring physicians who wished to view their images to physically sign out films from the radiology department's film library. Beyond the purposes of illustrating diagnosis to patients, family members, and consultants, these films were used for patient education and patient management. The Internet and its associated intranets increasingly have become the technologic basis for image management both within and outside the radiology department, as has been discussed in Chapter 5 on PACS and in Chapter 6 on teleradiology. As demonstrated, the Internet, due to its ubiquity, familiarity of use, and availability without incurrence of large installation costs, represents an ideal mechanism with which images can be made available to referring physicians. Most radiologists and referring physicians currently have Internet access; the addition of specialized software to enable them to receive images on their desktops can add to the power of the digital department.

A growing number of current PACS installations are now being specifically designed around Internet technology. As such, they are able to add Web-based solutions with relative ease. Central to the appeal of Web-based distribution is the fact that it allows any physician, whether at home or within the clinical setting, to use a personal computer as a virtual light box and view radiologic studies.

Early on, the visionaries in the PACS industry acknowledged the problem of image management and distribution. They encouraged engineers to approach radiology from an enterprise point of view to create a parallel structure in radiology with respect to the development of the electronic medical record. The guiding principle in system design was simply that there be an inherent ability to send images wherever alphanumeric medical information was sent. This task could be achieved by the flexible, integrated Web-based solution that would allow transmission of multiple types of information in textual, image, and video formats, among others.

Costs

There are other benefits to utilizing the WWW as the basis for image viewing outside the radiology department. First, the cost of primary interpretation workstations on the current UNIX platform can reach $70,000; these workstations are not a viable alternative for referring physicians who need to review radiology studies. While many vendors are moving toward cheaper, more conventional desktop systems to run workstation software, the majority of current installations still employ the UNIX solution.

Second, the current availability of the desktop PC as a patient care resource obviates the need for custom-designed image distribution channels. For example, the Partners HealthCare System, Boston (the parent corporation of the Massachusetts General Hospital and the Brigham and Women's Hospital) currently has approximately 30,000 PCs on the information systems network. During the deployment of our EPR solution and radiology image distribution system, this resource could be employed at no cost to the radiology department.

EMR: One Story

As with voice recognition, the experiences of others always help in illustrating pitfalls and benefits. The remainder of this chapter describes our experience at Massachusetts General Hospital (MGH) with the installation of an EPR system, an experience probably similar to that of other institutions. If you currently do not have an EPR solution at your institution, picture your hospital as you make your way through our installation.

A fully functional departmental PACS was installed in a component-based fashion at the Massachusetts General Hospital from 1996 through 1999. During the same 3-year time frame, the MGH Department of Information Sciences completed the creation of a clinical data repository (Figure 8-1), primarily for the purposes of electronic results reporting. The results encompassed primarily text-based result data recorded by the various departmental information systems already in place throughout the enterprise. These data were made available to the thousands of affiliated physicians throughout the network on thousands of personal computers using the electronic patient record system.

Over the course of our PACS installation, it became apparent that the system began to contain more and more critical imaging data. As the EPR effort rolled out throughout the enterprise and gained widespread acceptance, the need became apparent for the radiology department to electronically deliver not only our legacy text-based report results but also these critical image data. At that time, several methods of providing this necessary digital image transfer were investigated.

We implemented a WWW-based solution in 1995 as a part of our digital department initiative, since it was a solution that would allow the radiology department to automatically and cost-effectively maneuver radiology images to all clinicians. The growing popularity of the WWW over the past 5 years guaranteed a degree of familiarity with the client software. Additionally, this solution was easy to use and easy to install due to low support costs from the parent information systems (IS) group. The Web server solution could layer onto the basic system with coded access numbers, encryption, and VPN technology that enabled the radiology group to appropriately ensure security and patient confidentiality regardless of the referring physician's Internet access provider.

Getting to a Web-Based Solution

The Web solution, however, was not the first proposed solution. The first proposed solution involved the manipulation of image data in a similar fashion to textual data, with the ability to archive to systems such as CDR for later clinical retrieval. This approach was quickly rejected for several reasons. The primary exclusion criteria revolved around the problem that current CDR technology was not capable of expanding to the massive data requirements of medical images. Additionally, the engines behind Compact Disc Recordable (CDR) access applications had no mechanism for the display of medical image data on the client's computer.

Due to the shortcomings of the first solution, a second solution was quickly explored. It was proposed that images easily could be identified due to a unique identification (ID) in the DICOM header. This identifier would allow the EPR application to retrieve material from the departmental PACS. If images were too large to be contained on the CDR, the images could remain on the PACS and, through the use of DICOM unique identifiers, the CDR could forward requests to the PACS. These images then could be displayed to the client through a viewer application within the EPR. Again, several issues prevented this approach. First, the existing network infrastructure (a variety of bandwidths ranging from 10 Mbs shared to 100 Mbs switched) could not support the potential of thousands of requests for the transfer of minimally compressed medical image data (PACS 2:1 lossless JPEG). Second, the PACS could not support thousands of requests to its database server without serious performance degradation within the radiology department and without a cost to the work-flow efficiency of the radiologist. Finally, within the current iteration of the EMR client and within the departmental PACS, there did not exist a viewer application that was "thin" enough to execute on the thousands of enterprise-wide personal computers.

The elimination of these two options created the necessity to construct an image data repository (IDR) (Figure 8-1).

Image Data Repository

It quickly was decided that the IDR be an Internet-based system with the capability of DICOM communication that would include clinically acceptable images via a lossy image compression algorithm. It was preferred that expansion of the system would ultimately occur through a distributed architecture versus single-focused expansion of a main server. As performance requirements were initially defined, it was apparent that subsecond image access for potentially several hundred simultaneous users would require powerful back-end hardware and software.

At its core, the IDR essentially was a relational database and Internet Web server. The system communicated with the PACS via DICOM and was set as a storage class provider (SCP) to receive all image data that the PACs received from modalities. These image data then were wavelet compressed (at various compression ratios ranging from 10:1 to 20:1 depending on modality type) and stored in the database along with the DICOM header information (image type, series details, and user IDs) and the MRN and accession numbers that are received by the PACS from the radiology information system (RIS) during exam validation.

Prior to EPR integration, a stand-alone browser view application was written to support the decompression and display of these transmitted image data for clinical review. This application previously had been used as a viewer distinct from the EPR application physicians used to receive medical image data on hospital-wide PCs. Since the clinicians often were able only to provide medical record numbers or last names, a query mechanism was included in the browser application to search for image data based on any one of these parameters. It was this query mechanism that was used to interface the existing text-based EPR to the IDR.

During the review of radiology textual data within the EPR, the system is provided with the MRN and the accession number of the patient's examination being viewed. Using this information, the EPR with the IDR viewer is able to open a browser and populate with the associated images via a request to the IDR for the image data.

Caveats

Since the integration of the IDR client with the EPR, the IDR and EPR have served the clinical community without major technical problems. The unlimited concurrent user access to image data has been occurring for several years and appears to be without serious limitation to the clinical needs. As with any installation of this magnitude, there are several challenges and exceptions to this smooth operation. These are as follows:

1. Missing accession number: It often is the case that examinations are performed without knowledge of the patient's MRN (e.g., trauma patients with no identification). The images of these examinations can enter the PACs prior to accurate MRN data and be retained there until the RIS assigns the appropriate accession number. Without the accession number, however, the IDR application is not capable of retrieving the necessary image data.

2. IDR archive limitations: The most recent studies performed within the institution usually constitute the majority of clinical data requested. The image archive of the IDR, therefore, has been limited to maintain compressed image data for approximately 6 months. Any material requested that dates prior to 6 months from the current date is sent to another browser application that allows the user to request the data from the long-term PACS archive. As a request of this sort often can take extended lengths of time (depending on the current load on the PACS archive), the requesting user has the option to enter a pager number so that immediate notification may be made when the images are ready for viewing.

3. Workstation limitations: The addition of image display on thousands of end user workstations was without problem in a large portion of the installed user base within the enterprise. However, there were several personal computers that were being used for clinical review that were limited in their display capabilities. On many of these workstations, certain video modes were not capable of displaying medical image data acceptably, and it was deemed that the decision regarding the quality of the display should be the responsibility of the IDR client. If it was determined that the machine's video system was not capable of acceptable display, the images were not shown, and a message was displayed instructing the user to contact the help desk for upgrade options.

Hardware

We currently have multiple Web/intranet image servers as the default DICOM destination of over 20 digital modalities (CT, MRI, US, CR, DR, fluoroscopy). Each of the Web servers includes a Java-based interface to the radiology information system and a DICOM autorouter to storage devices as well as to the PACS. Incorporated into the Web-based solution is the use of a wavelet image compressor/decompressor that preserves compatibility with DICOM workstations and a server to distribute images throughout the enterprise.

These Web servers enable subsecond, on-demand, image distribution without any impact on our PACS resources, since the servers contain their own archives. A Redundant Array of Inexpensive Disks (RAID) solution currently in the hundred gigabyte range in each Web server, a storage solution that grows as prices decline, caches over 2 months of studies. The use of wavelet compression preserves the 12-bit data and allows interactive window/level and magnification control within common Web browsers, such as Netscape Navigator and Microsoft Internet Explorer. An encoded autolayout capability initially displays CR and digitized film at a reduced resolution to desktops with smaller screens while making full resolution available on demand.

There are software clients available who are able to utilize the HTTP protocol on nearly all platforms, not only Macintosh and PC. This allows the use of many types of integrated hardware in an EMR solution. Despite the wide availability of the physical connections to the Internet, the myriad of various software implementations—Java virtual machines, protocols, and scripting language interpreters—still often renders these platforms as unique as they were before the Internet. This becomes particularly true for radiology enterprise applications that involve medical image display.

Image Flow/Work Flow

Access to the image servers is available over the Web or intranet using Netscape Navigator or Internet Explorer. The minimal client resides on conventionally available PCs, typically 300 MHz Pentium PCs with 64 MB of RAM, with either Microsoft Windows 95/98 or Microsoft Windows NT, a TCP/IP stack, and a PPP connection to an Internet/intranet service provider. The wavelet compression method that the Web server solution uses will transmit the full 12-bit data set to the Web browser, allowing the user to interactively modify the window and level settings that specify the translation from 4,096 to 256 shades of gray. This wavelet plug-in is available for most major platforms, with other platforms accessing images using the JPEG format. The JPEG compression format, however, does not allow for interactive manipulation of the gray-scale transformation; the system automatically makes a guess at the proper window and level values based on an intelligent algorithm that utilizes the image data, the radiologic modality, and study description information.

Future Applications

Despite the ability to distribute images throughout the enterprise using Web server technology, certain issues still exist. The necessity of providing copies of radiologic studies performed to the patient remains a reality in every radiology department. Conventionally, film libraries have provided original films, on the condition that the recipient confirms their return.

Since one of the fundamental goals of the PACS is to reduce costs, patients will not be supplied with film-based copies. Providing images to patients in an electronic format obviates the need to print copies of films and ultimately creates savings to the operating budgets. An electronic distribution format (CD-ROM, DVD, etc.) also provides the patient with a permanent electronic copy of the radiologic studies performed in their health care management. Within the global health care system, additional savings can be achieved, since repeated radiologic studies can be eliminated.

The benefits of Web server utilization for image distribution stem from the ability to convert DICOM and RIS to Web-based data. The WWW allows the referring physician to receive text as well as images in a similar fashion without the need to learn different viewers to manipulate the data. In addition, this system allows the use of standard queries with familiar search-engine interfaces, eliminating the need for special training. The conventional browser is able to empower the referring physician to receive information from both electronic medical records systems and the PACS. Thus, the addition of Web servers to an electronic imaging effort bestows an added level of convenience and ease of use on clinicians. In the future, Web-based services will prove to be an essential component of the PACS by allowing complete elimination of film in CT, MRI, and ultrasonography.

Part IV
Resources

9
Radiology Websites

Portals	Journals/Publications
Teaching Files/CME	Magazines
Modalities	Divisons/Departments
Nuclear Medicine	Vendors
MRI	Book Vendors/Teaching Materials
Ultrasound	Associations/Centers
CT	Patient Resources

Portals

Auntminnie.com

Auntminnie.com serves as a complete information and resource site for radiologists, both practicing and in-training, as well as for other personnel affiliated with the practice of radiology. There are daily updates on news items, teaching cases, information about people in the radiology news, and discussion forums. Other resources provided include articles and forums about technology, education, markets, and the marketplace. Auntminnie.com offers services such as CME, setting up websites for practices, conference listings, and daily information fax services. An affiliated bookstore as well as ancillary services such as high-speed access and advertising that may interest some users are also available. Registration is required in order to use many of the site's features.

Dimag.com

Dimag.com provides a comprehensive daily update to the news in radiology. This website is an adjunct to the published monthly magazine that covers all topics in radiology practice. It also has links to special features including PACS, teleradiology, and MRI, among others. Access to webcasts (broadcasts) from RSNA as well as to past forums is available. This website provides a vast source of new information as well as archives of useful data.

Radcentral.com

Radiology Central is a resource for radiologists run by a radiologist—Gary Radner, Director of Neuroimaging, Childrens Hospital Los Angeles, and Assistant

Professor of Radiology, University of Southern California. This site provides links for medical news in both radiology and general medicine, cases of the week/month websites, organizations, and departments, as well as specialty and educational resources. This is a good website to start with if one also wants information about medicine in general.

Radinfonet.com

Radiology Info Net is a website with such resources for radiologists as online CME, cases, protocols, news, practice management information, and other information pertinent to the practicing radiologist. There are useful links to a conference calendar, expert opinions on subspecialty areas, and a forum for discussion with other radiologists.

Radiologist.com/comm1a.htm

Radiologist.com is a resource site for radiologists run by a radiologist. It exclusively includes links to sites that are pertinent to the radiologist, including radiology websites, educational resources, societies and journals, teleradiology, PACS, and DICOM, as well as specific modalities and subspecialties. This site is a good beginning resource to explore the world of radiology on the web.

Radiology.com/pacs

Radiology.com has secured the most coveted URL of all the portals. It was founded in 1989 and later acquired in 1997 by iWeb Corporation for corporate development. Radiologist.com servces as an application service provider (ASP) with services that enable digitized medical images to be stored, retrieved, and transmitted online through a central, web-based image repository called ImageBank™. This is not a resource portal to research other radiology websites.

Radiologyweb.com

Radiologyweb.com is a comprehensive site for radiologists, both practicing and in-training, with fact- and information-filled sections from "Insights and Impressions" to cases of the month. A CME, meeting finder, and job listings are included. The structure of this website is interesting in that it is commercially backed by an unrestricted grant from Bracco Diagnostics, has a team running the website, and is supported with educational material from an impressive list of individuals from Yale to Hong Kong. Registration is required to use most of the information available.

Education

Armed Forces Institute of Pathology: www.radpath.org
This website provides the course syllabus for the popular Radiologic Pathologic Correlation Course each studying doctor in the country takes during his/her residency. There is a wealth of knowledge with information ranging from the rarest bone tumors to common infections.

CHORUS, Medical College of Wisconsin: chorus.rad.mcw.edu
The Collaborative Hypertext of Radiology is a phenomenal resource with 1,100 index card pages covering all major entities in radiology. Salient and pertinent points are covered as a quick reference to remind or jog ones memory about rare diseases or differentials. The CHORUS collection is offered in a to-go version for palm pilots and other handheld devices.

CT is US: www.CTISUS.org
CT is US is a beautiful website with stunning visuals and content. There is information on protocols, teaching cases, and lectures on topics in CT imaging. Also included are updated protocols, particularly for multislice imaging, references, and a journal club. A medical illustration gallery that has amazing color illustrations of various pathological processes is present.

EUFORA: www.devolder.be/eufora/
Eufora.org allows access to the European Forum for Radiologists. This website contains a listserv that allows one to stay abreast of new communications from radiologists around the world. The main page also provides a link to www.thecybrary.com, a website run by Ncomed that provides resources to medical professionals in various disciplines.

A
Advanced Tools for Learning Anatomical Structure:
   http://www.med.umich.edu/lrc/Atlas/atlas.html
Amiga Radiologist: *http://www.octet.com/~mikety/index.html*
An Educational Resource, American Roentgen Ray Society:
   http://www.arrs.org/edu/
An Interactive Tutorial on Normal Radiology, Radiologic Anatomy:
   http://www.med.ufl.edu:80/medinfo/rademo/raintro.html
Anatomy-CID: *http://www.cid.ch/*
Anatomy Module List: *http://www.rad.washington.edu/anatomy/index.html*
Anatomy Teaching Modules:
   http://www.rad.washington.edu/anatomy/index.html
Armed Forces Institute of Pathology: *http://www.Afip.org*
Atlas of the Body, American Medical Association:
   http://www.ama-assn.org/ama/pub/category/7140.html

Atlas of Brain Perfusion SPECT:
http://brighamrad.harvard.edu/education/online/BrainSPECT/BrSPECT.html
Atlas of Myocardial Perfusion SPECT, BrighamRAD:
http://brighamrad.harvard.edu/education/online/Cardiac/Cardiac.html
ATS Radiology for Chest Physicians: CME Testing Modules:
http://www.vh.org/Providers/Simulations/ATS/ATS.html
AuntMinnie's Rad-Path Compendium!: *http://www.auntminnie.com*

B

Back Pain in Children: *http://www.vh.org/Providers/Textbooks/*
BackPainInChildren/BackPainChildren.html
Basics of MRI: *http://www.cis.rit.edu/htbooks/mri/*
Board Review Notes:
http://medicine.creighton.edu/radiology/Boardrevnotes.html
Body Teaching Files: *http://www.uhrad.com/ctarc.htm*
Brigham and Women's Hospital HMS (BrighamRAD):
http://brighamrad.harvard.edu

C

Caltech Radiation Safety Training and Reference Manual:
http://www.cco.caltech.edu/~safety/trm.html
Case of the Month, Brigham and Women's Hospital:
http://splweb.bwh.harvard.edu:8000/pages/comonth.html
Case of the Month, Department of Radiology, Nagasaki University:
http://www.med.nagasaki-u.ac.jp/radiolgy/case1.html
Case of the Week, Division of Diagnostic Imaging, University of Texas:
http://rpiwww.mdacc.tmc.edu/di/dicwdiag.html
Case of the Week, Rush-Presbyterian-St. Luke's Medical Center:
http://www.rad.rpslmc.edu/tf/cotw.html
Case Studies in Oral and Maxillofacial Radiology, Dalhousie University:
http://bpass.dentistry.dal.ca/casestudies.html
Cases for Nuclear Medicine, Tokai University:
http://www.gentili.net/TF98/39.htm
Cases from South Bank University:
http://www.sbu.ac.uk/~dirt/im0.html
The Chest XRAY: *http://www.chestx-ray.com/*
Chest X-Ray, Loyola University:
http://www.meddean.luc.edu/lumen/MedEd/medicine/pulmonar/cxr/cxr.htm
Children's Hospital of Birmingham, AL:
http://www.uab.edu/pedradpath/cases.html
CHORUS—Medical College of Wisconsin: *http://chorus.rad.mcw.edu/*
Clinical Nuclear Medicine, Loyola University:
http://lunis.lumc.edu/nucmed/tutorial/boneimg/

Clinical Teaching Case of Interest, Nuclear Medicine, University of Kansas:
   http://www.rad.kumc.edu/nucmed/clinical.htm
Colposcopy Atlas: *http://lib-sh.lsumc.edu/fammed/atlases/colpo.html*
Columbia-Presbyterian Medical Center: *http://cpmcnet.columbia.edu/*
Congenital Heart Disease on the Web:
   http://www.med.umn.edu/radiology/cvrad/chd/
Continuing Medical Education Testing Modules, Radiology for Chest
   Physicians Conference, American Thoracic Society:
   http://vh.radiology.uiowa.edu/Providers/Simulations/ATS/ATS.html
Correlapedia—Pediatric Imaging and Surgical Path:
   http://www.vh.org/Providers/TeachingFiles/CAP/CAPHome.html
Courseware for Microscopic, Radiologic, and Gross Anatomy:
   http://www.med.ufl.edu/medinfo/hamara/hamara.html
Creighton University: *http://www.creighton.edu*
CT Is US: *http://www.ctisus.org*
CyberAnatomy101:
   http://www.vislab.usyd.edu.au/gallery/vrml/tou/ingal/cyber_anatomy/

D
Dalhousie University: *http://bpass.dentistry.dal.ca/casestudies.html*
Debrecen, Hungary University Medical School—Online Neuropathology Atlas:
   http://www.neuropat.dote.hu/atlas.html
Diagnosis of Pulmonary Embolus:
   http://www.vh.org/Providers/Textbooks/ElectricPE/ElectricPE.html
Diagnostic Radiology, Internet Continuing Medical Education:
   http://www.cme.wisc.edu/fellow.html
Digital Anatomist Program:
   http://www1.biostr.washington.edu/DigitalAnatomist.html

E
ElectricLungAnatomy:
   http://www.vh.org/Providers/Textbooks/LungAnatomy/LungAnatomy.html
Eufora: *http://www.devolder.be/eufora/*
Experimental Radiology Teaching Files: *http://www.rad.swmed.edu/teach.html*

F
Fetal Echocardiography Gold: *http://www.fetalecho.com/*

G
Gaston Radiology: *http://www.gastonradiology.com/if_cases.html*

I
Indiana University: *http://www.iu.edu/*
Interesting Case of the Month, Section of Neuroradiololgy, University of
   California, San Francisco: *http://www.neurorad.ucsf.edu/case/index.html*

Interesting Case Review, Department of Radiology, Wayne State University:
  http://www.med.wayne.edu/diagRadiology/InterestingCase.html
Interesting Cases, Division of Radiologic Sciences, Wake Forest University:
  http://www.rad.bgsm.edu/radmain/htmls/cases/cases.html
Introduction to Clinical Medicine: Radiology, Virtual Hospital:
  http://www.vh.org/Providers/Lectures/icmrad/Opening.html
Introduction to Radiology, Michigan State University:
  http://kobiljak.msu.edu/CAI/RAD553/Title.html

J

Joint Fluoroscopy, University of Iowa:
  http://www.vh.org/Providers/Textbooks/JointFluoro/JointFluroHP.html
Jud Gurney's Chest X-ray Page: *http://www.chestx-ray.com/*

L

Laurie Imaging Center: *http://130.219.15.246/*
Let's Play PET: *http://laxmi.nuc.ucla.edu:8000/lpp/*
Levit Radiologic-Pathologic Institute: *http://rpi.mdanderson.org/levit/*
LUMEN—Indiana University: *http://www.indyrad.iupui.edu/rft*
Loyola University: *http://www.meddean.luc.edu/lumen/*
Lung Tumors: A Multidisciplinary Database, Virtual Hospital:
  http://www.vh.org/Providers/Textbooks/LungTumors/TitlePage.html

M

Madigan Army Medical Center:
  http://www.mamc.amedd.army.mil/mamc/mamcexthome.htm
Main Radiology Teaching File, University of Washington:
  http://www.rad.washington.edu/maintf/index.html
Martindale's Radiology:
  http://www-sci.lib.uci.edu/~martindale/MedicalRad.html
M.D. Anderson: *http://www.mdanderson.org*
MedPix: *http://rad.usuhs.mil/synapse/index.html*
Medshare, BrighamRAD:
  http://brighamrad.harvard.edu/education/online/tcd/tcd.html
MetaTextbook of Pediatric Radiology: *http://www.vh.org/Providers/*
  TeachingFiles/MetatextbookPedRad/MetaTBPedRad.html
Michael Tobin Radiology: *http://www.octet.com/~mikety/*
Monthly X-Ray Teaching Files, Emergency Medicine, Vanderbilt University:
  http://www.mc.vanderbilt.edu/vumcdept/emergency/xrhome.html
MRI Artifact Gallery:
  http://chickscope.beckman.uiuc.edu/roosts/carl/artifacts.html
MRI Teaching Modules, University of Pennsylvania:
  http://www.rad.upenn.edu/rrp/modules/modules.html
Multimedia and Learning, Levit Radiologic-Pathologic Institute:
  http://rpiwww.mdacc.tmc.edu/mmlearn/index.html

Multimedia Learning, University of Texas M.D. Anderson Cancer Center:
  *http://www.mdanderson.org/departments/LevitRPI/dIndex.cfm?pn=966962
  A6-3898-4FEE-8D128A057707CF3C*

N

Nagasaki University Hospital of Dentistry: *http://www.dh.nagasaki-u.ac.jp/rad/*
NetMedicine Radiology Library: *http://www.mdchoice.com/xray/xrx.asp*
Neuroradiological Teaching File, Laurie Imaging Center:
  http://www.laurie.umdnj.edu/New_Tango_App/index.html
Neuroradiology Section, Radiology Teaching File, University of North Carolina:
  http://sunsite.unc.edu/jksmith/UNC-Radiology-Webserver/Neuroradiology.html
Neuroradiology Teaching File, University of Colorado:
  http://www.uchsc.edu/sm/neuroimaging/tf_intro.htm
Neuroradiology Teaching Files, uhrad.com: *http://www.uhrad.com/mriarc.htm*
NLM Visible Human Project:
  http://www.nlm.nih.gov/research/visible/visible_human.html
Pediatric Thoracopedia:
  http://www.vh.org/Providers/TeachingFiles/TAP/Thoracopedia.html
Normal Radiologic Anatomy, Virtual Hospital: *http://www.vh.org/Providers/
  TeachingFiles/NormalRadAnatomy/Text/RadM1title.html*

O

Online Teaching Cases, Brigham and Women's Hospital, Harvard Medical
  School: *http://brighamrad.harvard.edu/education/online/tcd/tcd.html*
Online Teaching, Department of Radiology, University of California, San
  Francisco: *http://www.radiology.ucsf.edu/postgrad/multimedia/teaching_
  files.shtml*
Oral and Maxillofacial Radiology Teaching File, Nagasaki University:
  http://w3.dh.nagasaki-u.ac.jp/tf/

P

Paediapedia—Pediatric Imaging Encyclopedia:
  http://www.vh.org/Providers/TeachingFiles/PAP/PAPHome.html
Pediatric Imaging Case Files, University of Minnesota: *http://www.tc.umn.edu/
  nlhome/m122/hitex001/pedsimage/PCASELISTNEW.HTML*
Pediatric Radiology Case of the Month, New York University:
  http://www.gentili.net/TF98/64.htm
PediatricRadiology.com: Pediatric Imaging Digital Library:
  http://pediatricradiology.com/
Pediatric Radiology Files, Virtual Hospital: *http://indy.radiology.uiowa.edu/
  Providers/TeachingFiles/PedRadSecTF/PedRadSecTF.html*
Pediatric Radiology Teaching File, University of Iowa College of Medicine:
  *http://indy.radiology.uiowa.edu/Providers/TeachingFiles/PedRadSecTF/PedR
  adSecTF.html*
Penn State Universty: *http://www.psu.edu*

Association of Emergency Physicians' Home Page: *http://www.aep.org*
Professional Education, BrighamRAD:
  http://brighamrad.harvard.edu/education.html

R
Radiax Physicians Focus: *http://www.radiax.com/focus/index.htm*
RadioDB: *http://www.unipa.it/~radpa/RDB/*
Radiology Anatomy Project:
  http://www.med.ufl.edu/medinfo/rademo/raintro.html
Radiographic Anatomy 2002:
  http://www.rad.bgsm.edu/~dschwarz/ra2002web/ra2002home.htm
Radiographic Anatomy of the Skeleton, Michael L. Richardson, M.D.:
  http://www.rad.washington.edu/radanat/
Radiographic Anatomy of the Skeleton, University of Washington:
  http://www.rad.washington.edu/anatomy/
Radiologic Anatomy Browser, Uniformed Services University:
  http://rad.usuhs.mil/rad/rudinsky/homepage.html
Radiologic Anatomy Images, Emory University: *http://www.cc.emory.edu:*
  80/ANATOMY/Radiology/Home.Page.MENU.HTML
Radiologic Anatomy Interactive Quiz, Gold Standard Multimedia:
  http://www.gemedicalsystems.com/education/ceonline/gsmra.html
Radiology, Creighton University: *http://radiology.creighton.edu/*
Radiology Case Base, University of Kentucky: *http://fellow1.mri.uky.edu/*
Radiology Case Studies, DOD Telemedicine:
  http://www.matmo.org/pages/caseStudies/radiology/radiology.html
Radiology Case of the Week, Boston Veterans Affairs Medical Center:
  http://www.bumc.bu.edu/Departments/PageMain.asp?Page=1901&
  DepartmentID=73
Radiology Cases and Archive, Tulane University: *http://www.mcl.tulane.edu/*
  departments/Radiology/rad_home/recasarc/recasarc.html
Radiology Cases in Neonatology, University of Hawaii:
  http://www2.hawaii.edu:80/medicine/pediatrics/neoxray/neoxray.html
Radiology Cases in Pediatric Emergency Medicine, University of Hawaii:
  http://www2.hawaii.edu:80/medicine/pediatrics/pemxray/pemxray.html
Radiology CME, University of Kansas: *http://www2.kumc.edu/nucmed/*
Radiology Continuing Medical Education Programs, University of California
  San Francisco: *http://postgrad.radiology.ucsf.edu/*
Radiology Continuing Medical Education, Canberra Hospital:
  http://www.canberrahospital.act.gov.au/education/clinical%5Fschool/pg.htm
Radiology Education Foundation: *http://www.refindia.net/*
Radiology for Medical Students, Thomas Jefferson University:
  http://www.medmark.org/rad/rad2.html
Radiology Museum, South Bank University:
  http://www.sbu.ac.uk/~dirt/museum/museum.html

Radiology Postgraduate Education (CME), University of California, San
  Francisco: *http://postgrad.radiology.ucsf.edu*
Radiology Teaching File, Nagasaki University:
  http://www.dh.nagasaki-u.ac.jp/rad/tf/
Radiology Teaching File, University of Alabama, Birmingham:
  http://www.rad.uab.edu:591/tf/
Radiology Teaching File, University of California, Los Angeles:
  http://www.harbor-ucla-radiology.org/TeachingFile.htm
Radiology Teaching File, University of North Carolina: *http://sunsite.unc.edu/*
  jksmith/UNC-Radiology-Webserver/UNCRadTeachingFile.html
Radiology Teaching File, Wayne State University:
  http://www.med.wayne.edu/diagRadiology/TeachingFile.html
Radiology Teaching Files, Indiana University:
  http://www.indyrad.iupui.edu/rtf/
Radiology Teaching Files, University of Colorado:
  http://www.uchsc.edu/uh/radiology/teaching/index.html
Radiology Teaching Files, University of Michigan:
  http://www.rad.med.umich.edu/
Radiology Teaching Site, University of Toronto:
  http://www.utoronto.ca/imaging
Radiology Teaching, Central Middlesex Trust:
  http://www.sbu.ac.uk/~dirt/im0.html
Radiology Topics from GS collection, South Bank University:
  http://www.sbu.ac.uk/~dirt/museum/g-topics.html
Renal Transplant Imaging Tutorial:
  http:www.radiology.co.uk/xrayfile/xray/tutors/renaltx/ren.htm
Rush Presbyterian-St. Luke's Med Center: *http://www.rush.edu*

S
Scottish Radiological Society (The X-ray Files):
  http://www.radiology.co.uk/xrayfile/xray/index.htm
Shimane Medical University:
  http://www.shimane-med.ac.jp/IMAGE/Radiology.HTML
Silhouette Sign Review, Central Middlesex Hospital:
  http://www.sbu.ac.uk/~dirt/museum/rootsilh.html
Skiagram, site by Ian Maddison: *http://skiagram.com/*
South Bank University: *http://www.sbu.ac.uk/*
SUNY Stony Brook: *http://www.informatics.sunysb.edu/nysrs/rad/*
Synapse Web (Microscopic Neuroanatomy Atlases): *http://synapses.bu.edu/*

T
Teaching Cases, Department of Radiology, University of Texas, San Antonio:
  http://radiology.uthscsa.edu/rad/cases.htm

Teaching File, Departments of Pediatric Imaging and Pathology, Children's
    Hospital Birmingham, Alabama: *http://www.uab.edu/pedradpath/cases.html*
Teaching File, Joint Program in Nuclear Medicine, Harvard Medical School:
    http://www.jpnm.org
Teaching File Network Access Page, Mallinckrodt Institute of Radiology:
    http://gamma.wustl.edu/home.html
Teaching File, RadPa: *http://www.unipa.it/~radpa/tf.html*
Teaching Files, Baylor College of Medicine:
    http://www.bcm.tmc.edu/radiology/Cases/Cases.htm
Teaching Files, Department of Radiology, Michigan State University:
    http://www.rad.med.umich.edu/
Teaching Files, MRI Center, Bhatia General Hospital:
    http://www.mribhatia.com/
Teaching Files, Yale University:
    http://info.med.yale.edu/diagrad/teach_link.html
Teaching Media, University of California, San Francisco:
    http://www.radiology.ucsf.edu
Teaching Programs, Uniformed Services University:
    http://radlinux1.usuf1.usuhs.mil/rad/home/teach.html
Thoracic Imaging on the Internet:
    http://www.auntminnie.com/index.asp?Sec=ref&Sub=thi
Thoracic Radiology for Medical Students, University of Michigan:
    http://www.med.umich.edu/lrc/radiology/radio.html
Thoracopedia: An Imaging Encyclopedia of Pediatric Thoracic Disease,
    Virtual Children's Hospital: *http://www.vh.org/Providers/TeachingFiles/
    TAP/Thoracopedia.html*
Tulane University: *http://www.tulane.edu*
Tutorials, the X-ray Files:
    http://www.radiology.co.uk/xrayfile/xray/tutors/tuts.htm

U
Ultrasound Case of the Week, University of Alberta:
    http://www.ualberta.ca/~raddi/
Ultrasound Interesting Cases, University of California, San Francisco:
    http://ultrasound.ucsf.edu/USCases.html
Ultrasound Teaching File, University of Alberta:
    http://raddi.uah.ualberta.ca/~hennig/teach/teach.html
Uniformed Services University: *http://www.usuhs.mil/*
United Medical and Dental Schools: *http://www.umds.ac.uk/*
University of Alabama, Department of Radiology: *http://www.rad.uab.edu/*
University of Brescia: *http://www.unibs.it/~gasparo/neuro.html*
University of British Columbia: *http://wwwrad.pulmonary.ubc.ca/*
University of California Los Angeles: *http://www.ucla.edu/*
University of California San Francisco: *http://www.ucsf.edu*

University of Colorado HSC:
  http://www.uchsc.edu/uh/radiology/teaching/index.html
University of Colorado Health Sciences Center: *http://www.uchsc.edu/*
University of Colorado—Neuroradiology:
  http://www.uchsc.edu/sm/neuroimaging
University of Connecticut: *http://www.uconn.edu/*
University Diwan Chand Satyapal Aggarwal Imaging Research Centre:
  http://www.dcaimaging.org/quiz.htm
University of Iowa Department of Radiology: *http://indy.radiology.*
  uiowa.edu/Providers/ProviderDept/InfoByDept.Rad.html
University of Iowa Neuroradiology Library: *http://www.uiowa.edu/~c064s01/*
University of Iowa (Brain Dissection):
  http://www.vh.org/Providers/Textbooks/BrainAnatomy/BrainAnatomy.html
University of Iowa (Virtual Hospital):
  http://www.vh.org/Providers/ProvidersDept/InfoByDept.Rad.html
Michigan Department of Radiology: *http://www.rad.med.umich.edu/*
University of Michigan—ATLAS:
  http://www.med.umich.edu/lrc/Atlas/atlas.html
University of Minnesota Peds Imaging:
  http://www.tc.umn.edu/~hitex001/pedsimage/peds.html
University of North Carolina: *http://sunsite.unc.edu/jksmith/*
  UNC-Radiology-Webserver/UNCRadTeachingFile.html
University of Palermo: *http://www.unipa.it/~radpa.html*
University of Texas HSC San Antonio: *http://nuc-med-uthscsa.edu/*
University of Texas SW Medical Center: *http://www.rad.swmed.edu/teach.html*
University of Toronto: *http://www.utoronto.ca/imaging/*
University of Tübingen—Neuroassistant:
  http://134.2.176.106/Neuroassistant/index.html
University of Washington Department of Radiology:
  http://www.rad.washington.edu
University of Western Ontario: *http://radnuc.lhsc.on.ca/uwo/*
Unknown Case of the Week, LUNISweb:
  http://lunis.luc.edu/lunis/library/UNKNOWNCASEOFTHEWEEK.HTML
Uroradiology Tutor, Department of Radiology, Columbia University:
  http://cpmcnet.columbia.edu/dept/radiology/TUTORIAL/

V

Virginia Mason Med Center: *http://www.vmmc.org/radiology/vmrad.htm*
Virtual Brain:
  http://www.vh.org/Providers/Textbooks/BrainAnatomy/BrainAnatomy.html
Virtual Anatomy Project:
  http://www.nlm.nih.gov/research/visible/animations.html
Virtual Physics in Radiology Tutorials, Department of Radiology, Medical
  College of Wisconsin: *http://iago.lib.mcw.edu/medphys/learning.htm*

Virtual Radiological Case Collection:
http://radserv.med-rz.uni-sb.de/static/en/index.html
The Visible Embryo: *http://www.visembryo.com/baby/index.html*

W

Wake Forest University: *http://www.wfu.edu/*
Washington University School of Medicine Neuroscience Tutorial:
http://thalamus.wustl.edu/course/
Wayne State University Radiology Teaching File:
http://www.med.wayne.edu/diagRadiology/TeachingFile.html
Whole Brain Atlas: *http://www.med.harvard.edu/AANLIB/home.html*
World of the Thoracic Radiology, Korean Society of Thoracic Radiology:
http://www.medmark.org/korea2/korean2.html

X

X-ray Files: Teaching Radiology on the Internet:
http://www.gla.ac.uk/External/SRS/xrayfile/enter.htm
X-Ray Teaching Files, Vanderbilt University:
http://www.mc.vanderbilt.edu/vumcdept/emergency/xrhome.html

Y

Yale University: *http://info.med.yale.edu/diagrad/teach_link.html*
Yale University School of Medicine (Cranial Nerves):
http://info.med.yale.edu/caim/cnerves/

Modalities

Let's Play PET:
http://laxmi.nuc.ucla.edu:8000/lpp/shocked/lppshocked.html
Let's Play PET offers an online tutorial that covers much of the technology and
instrumentation behind the growing field of PET imaging. There is an overview
of PET as well as of subjects ranging from radioisotope production to PET trac-
ers and clinical applications of PET.

NMR Information Server: http://www.spincore.com/nmrinfo
The NMR information server was established in 1994 for the worldwide community of those interested in magnetic resonance. The NMR Information Server
provides magnetic resonance–related information services that include publishing news from around the world, articles, reports, reviews, photographs, and position announcements. Additionally, the NMR Information Server provides access to a Web-operated NMR Spectrometer. The WWW NMR Spectrometer can
be used for teaching, research, or service.

American Institute of Ultrasound in Medicine: www.aium.org
The AIUM website provides a host of information for the ultrasonographer from information about the *Journal of Ultrasound in Medicine* (*JUM*) to the education and research fund and consumer and provider information sites. It includes a search engine as well as up-to-date information about ultrasound products and meetings.

Nuclear Medicine

A

American College of Nuclear Physicians: *http://www.acr.org*
American Nuclear Society: *http://www.ans.org/*
American Society of Nuclear Cardiology: *http://www.asnc.org/*
American Counsel Users of Radioactive Isotopes: *http://www.acuri.com/*
Arizona Society of Nuclear Medicine: *http://www.ahsc.arizona.edu/azssnm/*
Associazione Italiana di Medicina Nucleare: *http://www.sameint.it/aimn/*
Australian and New Zealand Society of Nuclear Medicine:
   www.anzsnm.org.au

B

British Nuclear Medicine Society: *http://www.bnms.org.uk/*

C

Canadian Nuclear Association: *http://www.cna.ca/*
Canadian Nuclear Society: *http://www.cns-snc.ca/*
Cases Related to Nuclear Medicine, Tokai University:
   http://mfs.med.utokai.ac.jp/radiology/cases.html
Center For Positron Emission Tomography (CPET), University of Buffalo:
   http://www.nucmed.buffalo.edu/cpethm.htm
Centre for Positron Emission Tomography, Austin and Repatration Medical
   Centre: *http://www.austin.unimelb.edu.au/dept/PET*
Clinical Nuclear Medicine, Loyola University:
   http://lunis.luc.edu/nucmed/tutorial/boneimg/
Clinical PET Centre, Guy's and St. Thomas' Hospital:
   http://www-pet.umds.ac.uk/
Clinical Teaching Case of Interest, Nuclear Medicine, University of Kansas:
   http://www.rad.kumc.edu/nucmed/clinical.htm
Computer and Instrumentation Council, Society of Nuclear Medicine:
   http://gamma.wustl.edu/tf/caic.html
CYCERON Cyclotron BioMedical de Caen: *http://www.cyceron.fr/*
Cyclotron and PET Unit, Rigshospitalet, Copenhagen:
   http://www.pet.rh.dk/site/eng/
Cyclotron and RI Center, Nakamura Lab. Tohoku University:
   http://risun1.cyric.tohoku.ac.jp/

Cyclotron Unit, MRC CSC Hammersmith Hospital:
  http://www.cu.mrc.ac.uk/cyclotron_unit/contact_info.shtml/

D

Danish Society of Physiology and Nuclear Medicine: *http://www.dskfnm.dk/*

Department of Diagnostic Radiology and Nuclear Medicine, University of
  Western Ontario: *http://radnuc.lhsc.on.ca/uwo*

Department of Diagnostic Radiology and Nuclear Medicine,
  Rush-Presbyterian-St. Luke's Medical Center:
  http://www.rad.rpslmc.edu:80/

Department of Nuclear Medicine, University of Szeged:
  http://ss10.numed.szote.u-szeged.hu

Department of Nuclear Medicine, Gyeongsang National University Hospital,
  Korea: *http://www.ksnm.or.kr/english.shtml*

Department of Nuclear Medicine, Hokkaido University:
  http://radi.med.hokudai.ac.jp/index/html

Department of Nuclear Medicine, Kanazawa University:
  http://web.kanazawau.ac.jp/~med23/

Department of Nuclear Medicine Physics, Cedars-Sinai Medical Center:
  http://www.csmc.edu/medphys/

Department of Nuclear Medicine Technology, St. Vincent's Hospital and
  Medical Center: *http://www.nucmedicine.com/*

Department of Nuclear Medicine, State University of New York at Buffalo:
  http://www.nucmed.buffalo.edu

Department of Radiology and Radiological Sciences, Uniformed Service
  University of the Health Sciences:
  http://radlinux1.usuf1.usuhs.mil/rad/mainpage.html

Division of Nuclear Medicine, Children's Hospital, Boston:
  http://nucmedweb.tch.harvard.edu/

Division of Nuclear Medicine, Mallinckrodt Institute of Radiology,
  Washington University Medical Center: *http://gamma.wustl.edu/*

Division of Nuclear Medicine, New York University:
  http://nucmed.med.nyu.edu/rad.default.html

Division of Nuclear Medicine, Siriraj Hospital:
  http://www.mahidol.ac.th/mahidol/si/nmst.html

Division of Nuclear Medicine, St. Luke's-Roosevelt Hospital Center:
  http://www.wehealnewyork.org/professionals/residency/slr radiology.html

Division of Nuclear Medicine, State University of New York, Stony Brook:
  http://life.bio.sunysb.edu/biotech/ps/edu 95 96.html

Division of Nuclear Medicine, University of Arizona:
  http://www.ahsc.arizona.edu/azssnm

Division of Nuclear Medicine, University of British Columbia:
  http://www.1.stpaulshosp.bc.ca/

Division of Nuclear Medicine, University of Kansas:
  http://www.rad.kumc.edu/nucmed/

Division of Nuclear Medicine, University of Utah: *http://medlib.med.utah.edu/*
Dutch Working Group of Nuclear Cardiology and MRI:
  http://www.nuclcard.nl/index.htm

E
Emory University School of Medicine, Center for Positron Emission
  Tomography: *http://www.cc.emory.edu/RADIOLOGY/pet.html*
European Journal of Nuclear Medicine:
  http://www.link.springer.de/link/service/journals/00259/

G
Goulburn Valley Nuclear Medicine: *http://www.home.aone.net.au/ianalex/*

H
Hines VA School of Nuclear Medicine:
  http://lunis.lumc.edu/hines/school_info.html
HUG-IPNL PET Group: *http://dmnu-pet5.hcuge.ch/*

I
IEEE Transactions on Nuclear Science:
  http://www.ieee.org/organizations/pubs/transactions/tns.htm
Institute for Clinical PET (ICP): *http://www.icppet.org/*
Institute of Physics and Engineering in Medicine Electronic Journals:
  http://www.iop.org/journals/jnkubj
International Atomic Energy Agency (IAEA): *http://www.iaea.org/worldatom/*
International College of Nuclear Medicine Physicians:
  http://www.icnmp.edu.mx

J
Joint Program in Nuclear Medicine, Harvard Medical School:
  http://www.jpnm.org/
Journal of Nuclear Medicine Technology:
  http://www.snm.org/about/jnmt_order.html

L
Let's Play PET, University of California, Los Angeles:
  http://www.crump.ucla.edu/lpp
Lund Nuclear Data Service:
  http://nucleardata.nuclear.lu.se/nucleardata/nd.asp?page=Home

M
Medical PET Group—Biological Imaging, German Cancer Research Center:
  http://www.dkfz-heidelberg.de/pet/home.htm
My PET, Haluk Alibazoglu, M.D.: *http://www.ameripet.net/mypet.html*

N

National Council on Radiation Protection and Measurements, U.S.:
  http://www.ncrp.com/
National Nuclear Data Center, U.S.: *http://www.nndc.bnl.gov/*
Neuroradiology Section (Unknowns), Department of Defense, U.S.:
  http://www.matmo.org/pages/caseStudies/radiology/neuro/neuro.html
Nuclear Cardiology Department, Crawford Long Hospital:
  http://www.emory.edu/CRL/
Nuclear Energy Institute: *http://www.nei.org/*
Nuclear Engineering Department, University of Tennessee:
  http://www.engr.utk.edu/nuclear/
Nuclear Information System, Loyola University: *http://lunis.lumc.edu/lunis/*
Nuclear Medicine Communications Online:
  http://www.nuclearmedicinecomm.com/
Nuclear Medicine Imaging of the Gastrointestinal Tract, Virtual Hospital:
  http://www.vh.org/Providers/Textbooks/ElectricGiNucs/GINucs.html
Nuclear Medicine Media Book: *http://www.crump.ucla.edu/NM-Mediabook/*
Nuclear Medicine Research Council: *http://www.cbvcp.com/nmrc/*
Nuclear Medicine Review Manual:
  http://www.auntminnie.com/ScottWilliamsMD2/nucmed/contentsnucleartextb
  ook.htm
Nuclear Medicine Section, Radiology Teaching File, University of North
  Carolina: *http://sunsite.unc.edu/jksmith/UNC-Radiology-Webserver/*
  NuclearMedicine.html
Nuclear Medicine Section, University of Dundee:
  http://www.dundee.ac.uk/MedPhys/sections/NuclearMedicine.htm
Nuclear Medicine Technology Program, Cedar Crest College:
  http://www2.cedarcrest.edu/academic/bio/nmt/nmt.htm
Nuclear Medicine, Canberra Hospital: *http://xray.anu.edu.au/nucmed/*
Nuclear Medicine, Delaware Tech, Wilmington Campus:
  http://www.dtcc.edu/wilmington/nmt/
Nuclear Medicine, Medical Matrix:
  http://www.medmatrix.org/_SPages/Nuclear_Medicine.asp
Nuclear Medicine, Walter Reed Army Medical Center:
  http://www.wramc.amedd.army.mil/departments/nuclear/
Nuclear Medicine: Cases, Tokai University: *http://www.gentili.net/TF98/39.htm*
Nuclear Regulatory Commission, U.S.: *http://www.nrc.gov/*
Nuclear Society of Slovenia: *http://www.drustvo-js.si/index_eng.htm*
Nuclear and SPECT Imaging Teaching Files:
  http://www.uhrad.com/spectarc.htm
NUCMEDNET: *http://www.nucmednet.com/*

O

OECD Nuclear Energy Agency: *http://www.nea.fr/*
OSEM—Nuclear Medical Imaging:
  http://www.osem.server-web.com/OSEM.html

P

PET Center, Aarhus University Hospital: *http://www.pet.au.dk/*

PET Center, Wake Forest University Baptist Medical Center:
http://www.wfubmc.edu/pet/

PET Center, University of Zurich Hospital: *http://www-usz.unizh.ch/PET/*

PET Centre, Uppsala University: *http://www.pet.uu.se*

PET and Nuclear Medicine Department, Royal Prince Alfred Hospital:
http://www.cs.nsw.gov.au/rpa/pet/

PET Imaging Center, Biomedical Research Foundation:
http://www.biomed.org/pet.html

PET Imaging Center, University of Texas–Houston: *http://pet.med.uth.tmc.edu/*

PET Imaging Group, University of Aberdeen:
http://www.biomed.abdn.ac.uk/Research/PET/

PET Lab, Mount Sinai Medical Center:
http://www.mssm.edu/psychiatry/PETlab.shtml

PET Program, Paul Scherrer Institute: *http://pss023.psi.ch/index.html*

Pet Center Directory in North America: *http://www.snidd.org/pet_toc_hp.htm*

Physical Characteristics of Nuclear Medicine Images, Brigham & Womens'
Hospital, Department of Radiology:
*http://brighamrad.harvard.edu/education/online/physicis/MooreNM/
PhysCharacLesson.html*

Positron Emission Tomography Center, Children's Hospital of Michigan:
http://pet.wayne.edu/about.html

Positron Emission Tomography Center, University of Pittsburgh Medical
Center: *http://www.pet.upmc.edu/*

Positron Emission Tomography Laboratory, Massachusetts General Hospital:
http://neurosurgery.mgh.harvard.edu/pet-hp.htm

Positron Emission Tomography, University of California, Los Angeles:
http://www.nuc.ucla.edu/html_docs/frame_pet.html

Positron Laboratory, University of Geneva:
http://www.unige.ch/sciences/DPMC/positrons/home.html

Production of Medical Isotopes at Hanford:
http://www.cbvcp.com/nmrc/isotopes.html

R

Radioisotopes in Medicine, Uranium Information Center Ltd.:
http://www.uic.com.au/nip26.htm

Radiotherapy: *http://www.radiotherapy.com/*

S

Section of Nuclear Medicine, Loyola University: *http://lunis.lumc.edu/lunis/*

Section of Nuclear Medicine, University of Illinois:
http://www.uic.edu/com/uhrd/nucmed/homepage.htm

Servicio de Medicina Nuclear, Hospital Infanta Cristina:
http://www.audinex.es/~jirayo/

Society of Nuclear Medicine: *http://www.snm.org/*
Society of Nuclear Medicine: Computer and Instrumentation Council:
  http://gamma.wustl.edu/caic.html
Society of Nuclear Medicine, Southern California Chapter:
  http://gamma.wustl.edu/caic.html
Society of Nuclear Medicine, Taiwan: *http://www.snm.org.tw/*
Spanish Nuclear Medicine Society: *http://www.semn.es*

T

T-2 Nuclear Information Service, Theoretical Division of the Los Alamos
  National Laboratory, University of California: *http://t2.lanl.gov/*
Table of Isotopes: *http://www.wiley.com/legacy/products/subject/physics/toi/*
Table of the Nuclides, Jonghwa CHANG, Korea Atomic Energy Research
  Institute: *http://hpngp01.kaeri.re.kr/CoN/index.html*
Truku PET Centre: *http://www.utu.fi/med/pet*

U

UK-PET Special Interest Group: *http://www-pet.umds.ac.uk/UKPET/*

V

Virtual Nuclear Tourist—Nuclear Power Plants Around the World:
  http://www.nucleartourist.com

MRI

A

Acorn NMR Inc.: *http://www.acornnmr.com/*
Association of Managers of Magnetic Resonance:
  http://www.chem.yale.edu/~bangertr/ammrl/ammrl.html

B

Basics of MRI, Joseph Hornak:
  http://www.cis.rit.edu/htbooks/mri/
Beckman Institute for Advanced Science and Technology:
  http://www.beckman.uiuc.edu/research/mri.html
Biological NMR, University of Bristol:
  http://www.bch.bris.ac.uk/staff/pfdg/nmr.htm
BioMag Laboratory, University of Helsinki: *http://www.biomag.helsinki.fi/*
BioMagResBank: *http://www.bmrb.wisc.edu/*
Biomedical Magnetic Resonance Laboratory (BMRL), University of Illinois:
  http://bmrl.med.uiuc.edu:8080/info/brochure.html
Blue Hen NMR Complex, University of Delaware:
  http://www.nmr.udel.edu/nmr/info2/bhnmr.htm

C

CABM Protein NMR Spectroscopy Laboratory:
  http://www.nmr.cabm.rutgers.edu/
Cardiac MRI Teaching File: *http://www.cardiac-mri.com/*
Cardiac MRI Anatomical Atlas, University of Auckland:
  http://www.esc.auckland.ac.nz/People/Staff/Thrupp/cardiacMRatlas.html
Center for Advanced Magnetic Resonance Technology, Stanford University:
  http://www-radiology.stanford.edu/research/RR.html
Center for Interdisciplinary Magnetic Resonance:
  http://www.magnet.fsu.edu/science/cimar/
Center for Magnetic Resonance Research, University of Minnesota Medical
  School: *http://www.cmrr.drad.umn.edu/*
Center for Magnetic Resonance, The University of Queensland:
  http://www.cmr.uq.edu.au/
Center for MR-Guided Therapy, University of Minnesota:
  http://www.med.umn.edu/radiology/cmrgt/
Clinical Magnetic Resonance Society: *http://www.cmrs.com*
Computational Staining of Magnetic Resonance Brain Images, Caltech
  Computer Graphics Group: *http://www.gg.caltech.edu/brain/computational-
  staining.html*
CRS4–Medical Imaging: *http://www.crs4.it/*

D

Delft University: *http://www.twi.tudelft.nl*
Department of Magnetic Resonance, Gent University:
  http://mri2-gw00.rug.ac.be/
Division of Magnetic Resonance Research, Johns Hopkins University:
  http://mri2-gw00.rug.ac.be/

E

Emory University, Frederik Philips Resonance Research Center:
  http://www.emory.edu:80/RADIOLOGY/MRI/FPMRRCb.html
Enhanced NMR Periodic Table, Texas A&M University;
  http://www.chem.tamu.edu/services/NMR/periodic/
Erasmus Course on Magnetic Resonance Imaging: *http://emri-erasmus.org/*
European Chinese Society for Clinical Magnetic Resonance:
  http://www.ecscmr.de/
European Society for Magnetic Resonance in Medicine and Biology:
  http://www.medicon.cz/Ikem/Conferences/ESMRMB/EsmrmbInfo.html

F

FTNMR FID Archive, Pacific Lutheran University:
  http://www.chem.plu.edu/fid_archive/fid_archive.html
Functional MRI: *http://www.functionalmri.org/mainpage.htm*

Functional MRI Home Page, Massachusetts General Hospital:
http://www.nmr.mgh.harvard.edu/fMRI/fMRI.html
Functional MRI Research Laboratory, Beckman Institute:
http://www.beckman.uiuc.edu/research/funcmri.html

G

Gainesville VAMC MRI Home Page: *http://www.gentili.net/TF98/30.htm*
GAMMA, A General Approach To Magnetic Resonance Mathematical
    Analysis: *http://gamma.magnet.fsu.edu/*
GE Research: *http://www.crd.ge.com/*
Global links. NMR Research Group, Yale University:
    http://mri.med.yale.edu/links.html
Goal-Directed Magnetic Resonance Brain Micro-Imaging, Caltech Computer
    Group: *http://www.gg.caltech.edu/brain/cit_brain.html*

H

Hatch NMR Research Center: *http://www.hatch-ultra.cpmc.columbia.edu/*

I

International Society for Magnetic Resonance in Medicine:
    http://www.ismrm.org/
International Society for Magnetic Resonance in Medicine, British Chapter:
    http://www-ipg.umds.ac.uk/ismrm-bc/

J

Japan Society for Magnetic Resonance in Medicine:
    http://wwwsoc.nii.ac.jp//jmrm/
Joint NMR Group, Ludwig Institute/University College London, Joint NMR
    Laboratory: *http://www.biochem.ucl.ac.uk/bsm/nmr/index.html*
Journal of Magnetic Resonance: *http://www.academicpress.com/jmr*

L

Laboratory of NMR Microscopy, University of Trieste:
    http://www.univ.trieste.it/~micronmr/

M

Magin's Research Laboratory, fMRI, University of Illinois, Urbana
    Champaign: *http://mrel.beckman.uiuc.edu/fmri/index.html*
Magnetic Properties and Magnetic Resonance, Bulletin of the Chemical
    Society of Japan: *http://www.chemistry.or.jp/journals/bcsj/index.html*
Magnetic Resonance Group, University of Nottingham:
    http://www.magres.nottingham.ac.uk
Magnetic Resonance Department, University Hospital Gent in Belgium:
    http://mri2-gw00.rug.ac.be/

Magnetic Resonance Imaging Journal, Elsevier Science:
   http://www.elsevier.nl:80/inca/publications/store/5/2/5/4/7/8/
Magnetic Resonance Imaging for Computer Graphics, Graphics and
   Visualization Center: *http://www.gg.caltech.edu/sitevis/mri_research.html*
Magnetic Resonance Imaging and Spectroscopy Group:
   http://www.beckman.uiuc.edu/research/mri.html
Magnetic Resonance Imaging, Brigham and Women's Hospital:
   http://www.researchmatters.harvard.edu/program.php?program_id=30
Magnetic Resonance Imaging, HSTAT, NIH, U.S.:
   http://text.nlm.nih.gov/nih/cdc/www/66.html
Magnetic Resonance Imaging, University of Chicago:
   http://www-radiology.uchicago.edu/sections/mri.html
Magnetic Resonance Lab, State University of Syracuse: *http://139.127.65.86/*
Magnetic Resonance Lab, University of Virginia:
   http://ernst.chem.virginia.edu/
Magnetic Resonance Laboratory, University of California, San Francisco:
   http://picasso.ucsf.edu/
Magnetic Resonance Facility, University of Illinois:
   http://bmrl.med.uiuc.edu:8080/
Magnetic Resonance Microscopy of Embryos, Duke University Medical
   Center: *http://wwwcivm.mc.duke.edu/civmPeople/SmithBR/brs.html*
Magnetic Resonance of New Jersey:
   http://www.drused.com/trade/aa015736.html
Magnetic Resonance Periodic Table, Biomedical Magnetic Resonance
   Laboratory and The University of Illinois:
   http://bmrl.med.uiuc.edu:8080/MRITable/
Magnetic Resonance Safety Site: *http://kanal.arad.upmc.edu/mrsafety.html*
Magnetic Resonance Sites Worldwide, Jonathan Callahan, University of
   Washington: *http://btcpxx.che.uni-bayreuth.de/NMR/nmr_groups.html*
Magnetic Resonance Spectroscopy and Methodology, University of Bern:
   http://ubecx01.unibe.ch/dkf1/amsm/index.htm
Magnetic Resonance, University of Washington:
   http://www.rad.washington.edu/
Medical Imaging, Yonsei University Biomedical Computer Lab:
   http://yimit.yonsei.ac.kr/MedicalImaging.key.htm
Metabolic Magnetic Resonance Research and Computing Center, University of
   Pennsylvania: *http://www.mmrrcc.upenn.edu/*
MR Angiography: *http://www.mrprotocols.com/*
MR Tutor Project, University of Sussex, Brighton:
   http://www.cogs.susx.ac.uk/users/mike/rad/mrtutor.html
MR-Center, Sintef, Trondheim, Norway: *http://www.mr.sintef.no/*
MRI Artifact Gallery:
   http://bmrl.bmrf.uiuc.edu:8080/mriartgallery/artifacts.html
MRI Center-Bhatia General Hospital, Mumbai: *http://www.mribhatia.com/*

MRI Center, University of Wisconsin, Madison:
http://www.ozzieweb.net.au/medical/radiology.htm
MRI Education Foundation: *http://www.mrieducation.com*
MRI in Heart and Circulation, Graham Wright, Ph.D., University of
Toronto/Sunnybrook Health Science Centre:
http://www.sunnybrook.utoronto.ca:8080/~gawright/menu_mr_nf.html
MRI of Hippocampus in Incipient Alzheimer's Disease, University of Kuopio:
http://www.uku.fi/laitokset/neuro/37the.htm
MRI Teaching Modules, University of Pennsylvania:
http://www.rad.upenn.edu/rrp/modules/modules.html

N
National High Magnetic Field Laboratory (NHMFL), Florida State University:
http://www.magnet.fsu.edu/
National Magnetic Resonance Facility at Madison:
http://www.nmrfam.wisc.edu/
Nijmegen-Amsterdam High Field Magnet Laboratory (HFML):
http://www-hfml.sci.kun.nl/hfml/
NMR and MRI Web Sites, Dalhousie University:
http://bpass.dentistry.dal.ca/mri.html
NMR Center, Massachusetts General Hospital:
http://www.nmr.mgh.harvard.edu/
NMR Center, University of Texas Medical Branch at Galveston:
http://www.nmr.utmb.edu/
NMR Centre, University of Guelph: *http://nmr.uoguelph.ca/*
NMR Concepts: *http://chemnt1.chm.uri.edu/nmr/*
NMR Home page, Edinburgh University:
http://www.chem.ed.ac.uk/Welcome.html
NMR Home Page, University of Cambridge Chemical Laboratory:
http://www-methods.ch.cam.ac.uk/meth/nmr.html
NMR Home Page, University of Potsdam:
http://www.chem.uni-potsdam.de/englisch/index.html
NMR Imaging Laboratory, University of Texas, Austin:
http://www.pe.utexas.edu/Dept/Labs/MRI/mri.html
NMR Imaging Laboratory, University of Tsukuba:
http://mrlab.bk.tsukuba.ac.jp/
NMR Information Server: *http://www.spincore.com/nmrinfo/*
NMR Lab, Russia: *http://www.nmr.ru*
NMR Research Center, Dartmouth Hitchcock Medical Center:
http://www.dartmouth.edu:80/www/dms/nmrbrl/
NMR Lab, Utsunomiya University: *http://mri.is.utsunomiya-u.ac.jp/*
NMR Research Group, Yale University: *http://mri.med.yale.edu/index.html*
NMR Research Unit, University College London: *http://www.ucl.ac.uk/CFN/*
NMR Spectroscopy, Imperial College of Science, Technology and Medicine:
http://www.ch.ic.ac.uk/local/organic/nmr.html

NMR Spectroscopy, NIH, U.S.: *http://www.nih.gov/sigs/SBC/nmr/cover.html*
NMR Spectroscopy, University of Oslo:
  http://www.kjemi.uio.no/~bjornp/Phys-NMR-hjemme.html
NMR Unit, University of Edinburgh:
  http://www.univ-lille1.fr/lcom/RMN2D/menu_rmn/index_us.htm
NMR WWW Server, European Molecular Biology Laboratory:
  http://www.nmr.embl-heidelberg.de/
NMR, Cambridge Center for Molecular Recognition (CCMR) Biomolecular
  NMR Facility: *http://www-ccmr-nmr.bioc.cam.ac.uk/*
NMR, Widener University: *http://science.widener.edu/svb/nmr/nmr.html*
NMRL, University of Illinois, Chicago:
  http://ditto.rrc.uic.edu/SERVICES/NMRL/
NMR, University of Macquarie: *http://www.chem.mq.edu.au/nmr.html*
NMRWeb, University of York: *http://www.york.ac.uk/depts/chem/services/nmr/*
NMR Group, University of Groningen: *http://www.chem.rug.nl/nmr/*
NMR Lab, University of Kansas: *http://www.chem.ukans.edu/anylresc/nmr/*
NMR Laboratory, University of Ferrara:
  http://www2.unife.it.chimica_nmr/index.htm
Nuclear Magnetic Resonance, University of Florida:
  http://micro.ifas.ufl.edu/nmr.html

O

Ohio State University: *http://medicine.osu.edu/rad/*
Overseas Chinese Magnetic Resonance Association (OCMRA):
  http://www.emory.edu/NMR/OCMRA/prod01.htm
Oxford Center for Functional Magnetic Resonance Imaging of the Brain:
  http://www.fmrib.ox.ac.uk/

P

Pediatric Orthopedic MRI, William A. Mize M.D., University of Minnesota:
  http://www.tc.umn.edu/nlhome/m122/hitex001/pedsimage/pdorthmr.html

R

Radiological Society of North America, Inc., Education Portal:
  http://www.rsna.org/education/launchpad/nuclear.html
Renal MRA, University of Michigan: *http://ej.rsna.org/ej3/0091-
  98.fin/index.html*
Rock NMRI (Nuclear Magnetic Resonance Imaging) Home Page, University
  of Texas at Austin: *http://www.pe.utexas.edu/Dept/Labs/MRI/mri.html/*

S

Safety for Nuclear Magnetic Resonance:
  http://mriris.rockefeller.edu/safety.html
SISCO/Varian Users Group: *http://bmrl.med.uiuc.edu:8080/SISCO/*
Society of Cardiovascular Magnetic Resonance (SCMR): *http://www.scmr.org/*

Society of Computed Body Tomography and Magnetic Resource:
  http://www.scbtmr.org
Solid State NMR Group, University of Laval Chemistry Department:
  http://www.chm.ulaval.ca/
Solid State NMR Lab, University of Nebraska at Lincoln:
  http://chem-harbison.unl.edu/homepage.html
Spectroscopy, Wilson Group, University of California, San Diego:
  http://www-wilson.ucsd.edu/education/pchem/spectroscopy/
Stereotactic MRI Brain Map of Japanese Monkey, Nihon University, FTP:
  ftp://ftp.nc.nihon-u.ac.jp/pub/data/MRIMonkeyHead/
Study the Structure of the Brain by MRI, Hanover College:
  http://psych.hanover.edu/Krantz/neural/021.html

T

Teaching Files, MRI Center, Bhatia General Hospital:
  http://www.mribhatia.com/
Tomographie Positron (TOPO), Universit Catholique de Louvain:
  http://topo.topo.ucl.ac.be/

U

UCSF MR Lab; *http://picasso.ucsf.edu/*
University of Alabama Birmingham: *http://depts.*
  washington.edu/chemnmr/Pencil_etc/PENCIL/Pencil_home_page.html
University of Chicago: *http://www.mri.uchicago.edu/*
University of Illinois: *http://bmrl.med.uiuc.edu:8080/*
University of Kent: *http://ramsey.chem.ualberta.ca/wwwnmr2.html*
University of Leeds—CoMIR: *http://www.comp.leeds.ac.uk/comir/comir.html*
University of Minnesota: *http://www.cmrr.drad.umn.edu*
University of Queensland: *http://www.cmr.uq.edu.au*
University of Texas at Arlington: *http://www.uta.edu*
University of Texas Southwestern:
  http://www.swmed.edu/home_pages/rogersmr

V

Varian NMR: *http://www.mri.jhu.edu/mri_sites.html*
Varian/SISCO MRI Users Group: *http://bmrl.med.uiuc.edu:8080/SISCO/*

W

Wageningen NMR Center, Wageningen Agricultural University:
  http://gcg.tran.wau.nl/wnmrc/wnmrc.html
WebSpectra—Problems in NMR and IR Spectroscopy:
  http://www.chem.ucla.edu/~webspectra/

Y

Yale NMR Research Group: *http://mri.med.yale.edu:80/*

Ultrasound

3D Ultrasound Resource, Bernard:
   http://www.cs.uwa.edu.au/~bernard/us3d.html

A

Acoustical Society of America: *http://asa.aip.org/*
Acuson Clinical Resources: *http://www.acuson.com/cme/index.htm*
American Endosonography Club: *http://www.duke.edu/eus/*
American Institute of Ultrasound in Medicine: *http://www.aium.org*
American Registry of Diagnostic Medical Sonographers:
   http://www.ardms.org/
American Society of Echocardiography: *http://asecho.org*
AmnioNet: *http://www.amnionet.com/*
Arizona Society of Echocardiography:
   http://aztec.asu.edu/medical/azse/azse0.html
ATL Reference Library: *http://www.kent.edu/*
Australian Institute of Ultrasound: *http://www.aiu.edu.au/*
Australian Society for Ultrasound in Medicine:
   http://www.asum.com.au/open/home.htm

B

Beth Israel Hospital:
   http://rudiology.bidmc.harvard.edu/about/frameset_info.html
Biomedical Engineering and Ultrasound diagnosis: *http://www.drgdiaz.com/*
Biomedical Ultrasonics Laboratory, University of Michigan:
   http://bul.eecs.umich.edu/
Biosound Esaote Ultrasound: *http://www.biosound.com/*
Burwin Institute of Diagnostic Medical Ultrasound: *http://www.Burwin.com*

C

Center for Medical Ultrasound, Bowman Gray School of Medicine:
   http://www.bgsm.edu/bgsm/ultrasound/
Center for Prenatal Diagnosis: *http://www.cpdx.com/cpdx/cntr.htm*

D

Diagnostic Ultrasound, Dr. Gonzalo Diaz: *http://www.drgdiaz.com/*
Diagnostic Ultrasound Imaging in Pregnancy, NIH, U.S.:
   http://text.nlm.nih.gov/nih/cdc/www/41cvr.html
Diagnostic Ultrasound, University of California San Francisco Medical Center:
   http://ultrasound.ucsf.edu/

E

E-chocardiography Journal: *http://www2.umdnj.edu/~shindler/echo.html*
Endoscopic Ultrasonography: *http://www.eus-online.org/*

Endosonography Endoscopic Ultrasound: *http://www.duke.edu/eus/*

Estimation of Blood Velocities Using Ultrasound. A Signal Processing Approach.: *http://www.es.oersted.dtu.dk.staff/jaj/book.html*

European Federation of Societies for Ultrasound In Medicine and Biology: *http://www.efsumb.org/*

European Journal of Ultrasound: *http://www.elsevier.nl:80/locate/estoc/09298266*

F

Fetal 3D Imaging, University College London: *http://www.medphys.ucl.ac.uk/mgi/fetal/*

Fetal Echocardiography Gold: *http://www.fetalecho.com/*

Fetal Sonography, Terry J DuBose: *http://www.io.com/~dubose/fs.html*

Fetal.Com: *http://www.fetal.com*

The Fetus: *http://www.thefetus.net*

Fetus.net: *http://www.thefetus.net/*

G

Gulfcoast Ultrasound Institute: *http://www.gcus.com/*

I

International Breast Ultrasound School: *http://www.ibus.org/*

Internet Fetal Echocardiography: *http://www.fetalecho.com/*

J

Jefferson Ultrasound Research and Education Institute: *http://jeffline.tju.edu/CWIS/DEPT/Ultrasound/JUREI/index.html*

Joseph Woo—Obstetrical Ultrasound: *http://www.ob-ultrasound.net*

Journal of Sound and Vibration: *http://www.apnet.com/www/catalog/sv.htm*

Journal of Ultrasound in Medicine: *http://www.jultrasoundmed.org/*

JS Spectromed: *http://www.spectromed.com/TIT_ENG.HTM*

L

Laboratory For Ultrasonics, University of Washington: *http://ultrasonics.wustl.edu/*

M

Medical and Scientific Information Online: *http://www.cpdx.com*

Musculoskeletal Ultrasound Society: *http://musoc.com/*

O

OB-GYN Ultrasound Online: *http://www2.ultrasoundedu.com/ultrasoundedu*

Online CME Courses, GE Ultrasound: *http://www.gemedicalsystems.com/rad/us/education/msucme.html*

P

Platypus—Prenatal Ultrasound Abnormality: *http://www.comnet.ca/~tki/*
Prenatal Diagnosis: *http://www.fetal.com*

S

Shimane University: *http://www.shimane-med.ac.jp/IMAGE/UStext/*
   normal-ustext.html
Society of Diagnostic Medical Sonographers: *http://www.sdms.org/*
Society of Radiologists in Ultrasound: *http://www.sru.org/*
Sonography Sources: *http://www.gl.umbc.edu/~mccormac/index.htm*
St. Paul's Hospital: *http://wwwrad.pulmonary.ubc.ca/StPaulsRadiol.html*
State of the Art Ultrasound: *http://www.drgdiaz.com/*
Stradivaius Project Summary, Cambridge University:
   http://svr-www.eng.cam.ac.uk/Research/Projects/Stradivarius/

T

Thomas Jefferson University:
   http://jeffline.tju.edu/CWIS/DEPT/Ultrasound/JUREI/index.html

U

ULTRANET: Ultrasound Technology:
   http://www.vltebsk.net/ultrasound/ultranet.htm
Ultrasound Artifacts:
   http://www1.stpaulshosp.bc.ca/stpaulsstuff/USartifacts.html
Ultrasound, Beth Israel Deaconess Medical Center East Campus:
   http://radiology.bidmc.harvard.edu/kinds_of_exams/ultrasound/
   ultrasound.html
Ultrasound Case Hotlist:
   http://home.earthlink.net/~terrass/radiography/medradhome.html
Ultrasound Case of the Week, University of Alberta:
   http://www.ualberta.ca/~raddi/ultrasnd/
Ultrasound Diagnosis: *http://www.drgdiaz.com/index.shtml*
Ultrasound Educational Press: *http://www2.ultrasoundedu.com/ultrasoundedu/*
Ultrasound Lab, University of Vienna:
   http://www.bmtp.akh-wien.ac.at/people/kollch1/home.html
Ultrasound in Obstetrics and Gynecology:
   http://obg.med.wayne.edu/ISUOG/home.htm
Ultrasound and Other Prenatal Diagnostic Tests, Stanford University:
   http://www.stanford.edu/~holbrook/
Ultrasound Physics, University of London:
   http://www.icr.ac.uk/physics/Ultrasound/Ultrasound-main.htm
Ultrasound in Pregnancy, NIH, U.S.:
   http://text.nlm.nih.gov/nih/cdc/www/41cvr.html
Ultrasound Research Laboratory, Mayo Clinic:
   http://www.mayo.edu/ultrasound/ultrasound.html

Ultrasound Review: *http://www.usreview.com.au/*
Ultrasound Section, Radiology Teaching File, University of North Carolina:
 http://sunsite.unc.edu/jksmith/UNC-Radiology-Webserver/Ultrasound.html
Underwater Acoustics and Medical Ultrasonics Group, University of Bath:
 http://www.bath.ac.uk/~pyscmd/acoustics/
University of Alberta: *http://www.ualberta.ca/~raddi/*
University of California San Francisco: *http://ultrasound.ucsf.edu*
University of Iowa—Liver Segmental Anatomy:
 http://everest.radiology.uiowa.edu/nlm/app/livertoc/liver/ultrasnd.html
University of Washington: *http://www.rad.washington.edu*

W
World Federation of Ultrasound in Medicine and Biology:
 http://www.wfumb.org/

CT
CTIS US.org: *www.ctisus.org*
Journal of Computer Assisted Tomography: *http://www.rad.wfubmc.edu/jcat/*

Journals/Publications

ACR Materials and Publications: www.acr.org/publications/mnp
The ACR materials and publications Web site provides the resources to acquire many of the documents that govern standards by which we practice radiology. These cover, among other topics, self-evaluation, practice management, and quality control.

Radiographics: http://radiographics.rsnajnls.org/
Radiographics provide an online resource of the popular journal. This Web site offers archives of past issues as well as information on upcoming issues. There is an online CME option as well as a search engine for information in the journal.

Radiology: http://www.rsna.org/publications/rad/index.html
The radiology Web site of the RSNA provides online access to members to the "gray" journal. It provides PDF versions of all articles published in Radiology as well as full-text searching, interjournal links to other radiology journals (as well as to all other journals) online with HighWire Press, links to PubMed, and e-mail notification of future tables of content.

A
The ABR Examiner: *http://www.theabr.org/examiner.htm*
AJNR—American Journal of Neuroradiology: *http://www.ajnr.org/*

Abdominal Imaging:
http://link.springer.de/link/service/journals/00261/index.htm
ACR Materials and Publications: *http://www.acr.org/publications/mnp/*
Acta Radiologica:
http://www.blackwellmunksgaard.com/tidsskrifter.nsf/a3b40ef0ca9b8d86c125
6a160050049f/d3e60879cc10c093c1256a1700507566?OpenDocument
American Journal of Neuroradiology: *http://www.asnr.org/ajnr/*
American Journal of Roentgenology: *http://www.arrs.org/ajr/*
Applied Radiation and Isotopes: *http://www.elsevier.com/locate/apradiso*
Applied Radiology: *http://www.appliedradiology.com*
Australasian Radiology: *http://www.blackwell-science.com/*
products/journals/xaura.htm

B

Basic Imaging Lectures: *http://medicine.creighton.edu/radiology/index.html*
British Journal of Radiology: *http://bjr.birjournals.org/*

C

Canadian Association of Radiologists Journal:
http://www.cma.ca/cma/common/displayPage.do?pageId=/staticContent/HTML/
N0/l2/carj/index.htm
Cancer Detection and Prevention: *http://www.cancerprev.org/*
CardioVascular and Interventional Radiology:
http://link.springer.de/link/service/journals/00270/index.htm
CHORUS—Collaborative Hypertext of Radiology: *http://chorus.rad.mcw.edu/*
Clinical Imaging: *http://www.elsevier.com/locate/clinimag*
Clinical Nuclear Medicine: *http://lww.com/store/products?0363-9762*
Clinical Positron Imaging:
http://www.sciencedirect.com/science?_ob=JournalURL&_issn=10950397&
_auth=y&_acct=C000050221&_version=1&_urlVersion=0&_userid=10&
md5=81546d281e6fc7df25e7ca8a765b00c3
Clinical Radiology: *http://www.harcourt-international.com/journals/crad*
Computerized Medical Imaging and Graphics:
http://www.elsevier.com/locate/compmedimag
Concepts in Magnetic Resonance:
http://www.interscience.wiley.com/jpages/1043-7347/
Contemporary Diagnostic Radiology:
http://www.bbk.ac.uk/fce2001/short/psycholshort.htm

D

Dentomaxillofacial Radiology: *http://www.naturesj.com/dmfr/*
Diagnostic Imaging: *http://www.dimag.com/*
Diagnostic Imaging Magazine Online: *http://www.dimag.com/*

E

E-chocardiography Journal: *http://www2.umdnj.edu/~shindler/echo.html*

Electronic AJR: *http://www.arrs.org/ajr/*

European Journal of Nuclear Medicine:
http://link.springer.de/link/service/journals/00259/index.htm

European Journal of Radiology: *http://www.elsevier.com/locate/ejrad*

European Journal of Ultrasound: *http://www.elsevier.com/locate/ejultrasou*

European Radiology:
http://link.springer.de/link/service/journals/00330/index.htm

European Radiology Online Database: *http://www.eurorad.org/*

H

High-Quality Mammography: Information for Referring Providers:
http://text.nlm.nih.gov/ftrs/pick?ftrsK50&collect5ahcpr&dbName5mamq

Human Brain Mapping: *http://www.interscience.wiley.com/jpages/1065-9471/*

I

Imaging Online: *http://imaging.birjournals.org/*

Indian Journal of Radiology and Imaging: *http://www.ijri.org/*

IEEE Transactions on Medical Imaging: *http://www.ieee-tmi.org/*

The International Journal of Cardiac Imaging:
http://www.wkap.nl/journalhome.htm/0167-9899

International Journal of Radiation Biology:
http://www.tandf.co.uk/journals/titles/09553002.html

International Journal of Radiation Oncology Biology Physics:
http://www.elsevier.com/locate/ijrobp

Investigative Radiology: *http://lww.com/store/products?0020-9996*

J

Japanese Journal of Magnetic Resonance in Medicine:
http://wwwsoc.nii.ac.jp/jmrm/abstract/abstracts.html

Journal of Clinical Ultrasound: *http://www.interscience.wiley.com/jpages/0091-2751/*

Journal of Computer Assisted Tomography: *http://www.rad.bgsm.edu/jcat/*

Journal of Diagnostic Medical Sonography:
http://www.sdms.org/jdms/default.asp

Journal of Digital Imaging (A):
http://link.springer.de/link/service/journals/10278/

Journal of Digital Imaging (B): *http://www.scarnet.org/*

Journal of Electronic Imaging: *http://www.spie.org/web/journals/jei_home.html*

Journal of Image Guided Surgery: *http://www.interscience.wiley.com:83/cas/*

Journal of Labelled Compounds and Radiopharmaceuticals:
http://www.interscience.wiley.com/jpages/0362-4803/

Journal of Magnetic Resonance: *http://www.apnet.com/www/journal/mn.htm*

Journal of Magnetic Resonance Imaging:
  http://www.interscience.wiley.com/jpages/1053–1807/
Journal of Neuroimaging:
  *http://www.sagepub.co.uk/frame.html?http://www.sagepub.co.uk/
  journals/details/j0374.html*
Journal of Nuclear Medicine: *http://www.snm.org/about/jnm_order.html*
Journal of Radiological Protection: *http://www.iop.org/Journals/jr*
Journal of Real Time Imaging: *http://www.academicpress.com/rti*
Journal of Thoracic Imaging: *http://lww.com/store/products?0883-5993*
Journal of Ultrasound in Medicine: *http://www.jultrasoundmed.org/*
Journal of Vascular and Interventional Radiology:
  http://lww.com/store/products?1051–0443

M
Magnetic Resonance Imaging (A): *http://www.elsevier.com/locate/mri*
Magnetic Resonance Imaging (B):
  http://cpmcnet.columbia.edu/dept/radoncology/outside.html
Medical Image Analysis: *http://www.elsevier.nl/locate/medima/*

N
NeuroImage: *http://www.academicpress.com/ni*
Neuroimaging Clinics:
  *http://www2.us.elsevierhealth.com/scripts/om.dll/serve?action=
  searchDB&searchDBfor=home&id=cnim*
Neuroradiology: *http://link.springer.de/link/service/journals/00234/index.htm*
News, Radiology, Doctors Guide: *http://www.pslgroup.com/dg/radionews.htm*
Nuclear Medicine: *http://www.elsevier.com/locate/nucmed*
Nuclear Medicine and Biology: *http://www.elsevier.com/locate/nucmedbio*
Nuclear Medicine Communications: *http://lww.com/store/products?0143-3636*

O
On Line Textbook of Normal Ultrasound, Shimane Medical University:
  http://www.shimane-med.ac.jp/IMAGE/UStext/normal-ustext.html

P
Pediatric Radiology:
  http://link.springer.de/link/service/journals/00247/index.htm
Progress in Nuclear Magnetic Resonance Spectroscopy:
  http://www.elsevier.nl/locate/pnmrs

Q
Quality Determinants of Mammography, Agency for Health Care
  Policy and Research:
  http://text.nlm.nih.gov/ftrs/pick?ftrsK50&collect5ahcpr&dbName5mamc

R

Radiation and Environmental Biophysics:
http://link.springer.de/link/service/journals/00411/index.htm

Radiation Oncology Investigations:
http://www.interscience.wiley.com/jpages/1065-7541/

Radiation Research: *http://www.radres.org/contents.htm*

Radiation Therapist:
http://www.asrt.org/other_categories/about_asrt/radiation_therapist.htm

Radiographics: *http://radiographics.rsnajnls.org/*

Radiography: *http://www.harcourt-international.com/journals/radi/*

Der Radiologe: *http://link.springer.de/link/service/journals/00117/index.htm*

Radiologic Clinics:
http://www2.us.elsevierhealth.com/scripts/om.dll/serve?action=
searchDB&searchDBfor=home&id=crad

Radiology (A): *http://www.medwebplus.com/obj/18268*

Radiology (B): *http://www.rsna.org/publications/rad/index.html*

Radiology, Doctor's Guide: *http://www.pslgroup.com/dg/radionews.htm*

Radiology News, Doctor's Guide: *http://www.pslgroup.com/dg/radionews.htm*

Radiotherapy and Oncology (A): *http://www.elsevier.com/locate/radonc*

Radiotherapy and Oncology (B): *http://www.nucgang.org/*

RSNA EJ: *http://ej.rsna.org/*

S

Seminars in Interventional Radiology:
http://www.thieme.com/SID2045929072286/journals/pubid2048889311.html

Seminars in Musculoskeletal Radiology: *http://www.thieme.de/smr/*

Seminars in Nuclear Medicine: *http://www.us.elsevierhealth.com/*
fcgi-bin/displaypage.pl?isbn=00012998

Seminars in Radiation Oncology:
http://www2.us.elsevierhealth.com/scripts/om.dll/serve?action=
searchDB&searchDBfor=home&id=srao

Seminars in Radiologic Technology:
http://www2.seminarsinradiologictechnology.com/scripts/om.dll/serve?action=
searchDB&searchDBfor=home&id=srat

Seminars in Roentgenology:
http://www.thieme.com/SID1987257926699/journals/pubid2048889311.html

Seminars in Ultrasound, CT and MRI: *http://www.us.elsevierhealth.com/*
fcgi-bin/displaypage.pl?isbn=08872171

Skeletal Radiology: *http://link.springer.de/link/service/journals/00256/index.htm*

Solid State Nuclear Magnetic Resonance:
http://www.elsevier.nl:80/inca/publications/store/5/2/2/5/3/7/

Surgical and Radiologic Anatomy:
http://link.springer.de/link/service/journals/00276/index.htm

T

Techniques in Vascular and Interventional Radiology:
http://www2.us.elsevierhealth.com/scripts/om.dll/serve?action=searchDB&searchDBfor=home&id=tvir

Topics in Magnetic Resonance Imaging: *http://lww.com/store/products?0899-3459*

U

Ukrainian Journal of Radiology: *http://www.imr.kharkov.ua/journal/*

Ultrasonics Sonochemistry:
http://www.elsevier.com:80/inca/publications/store/5/2/5/4/5/1/

Ultrasound Educational Press, University of California, San Francisco:
http://www2.ultrasoundedu.com/ultrasoundedu/default.html

Ultrasound in Medicine and Biology:
http://www.elsevier.com/locate/ultrasmedbio

Ultrasound in Obstetrics and Gynecology:
http://obg.med.wayne.edu/ISUOG/home.htm

Ultrasound Quarterly: *http://lww.com/store/products?0894-8771*

Ultrasound Review: *http://www.usreview.com.au*

Magazines

PACSweb: http://www.dimag.com/pacsweb/index.shtml
The PACSweb site is an information archive provided by the publishers of Diagnostic Imaging magazine. Supported by AGFA, an industry leader in the PACS arena, PACSweb provides valuable articles, discussions, and forums about all aspects of PACS.

Decisions in Imaging Economics: www.imagingeconomics.com
This website provides an online version, with archive searching capabilities, of the popular paper-based magazine. Focusing on economics in radiology, this Web site also provides links to special project supplements published by the magazine as well as a calendar and media kits for interested parties.

D

Decisions in Imaging Economics: *http://www.imagingeconomics.com/*

Diagnostic Imaging Archive: *http://www.diagnostic-imaging.com/search.shtml*

Diagnostic Imaging Asia Pacific Magazine:
http://www.diagnosticimaging.com/magazines/asia_pacific/

Diagnostic Imaging Europe Magazine:
http://www.diagnosticimaging.com/magazines/europe/

Diagnostic Imaging Magazine: *http://www.dimag.com*

H
Healthcare Informatics: *http://www.healthcare-informatics.com/*

I
Imaging Online: *http://dspace.dial.pipex.com/town/parade/ad828/*

P
PACS and Networking News: *http://www.pacsnews.com*
PACSweb: *http://www.dimag.com/pacsweb/index.shtml*

T
Telehealth: *http://www.telehealthmag.com/*

Divisions/Departments

Brighamrad, Department of Radiology, Brigham and Women's Hospital: http://brighamrad.harvard.edu
BrighamRAD provides a host of information, not only about the world-famous radiology department, but also links to educational resources for both patients and radiologists. Additionally, there are links to the Harvard Medicine School and affiliated organizations. Interesting areas include cutting edge research being conducted at the institution.

Creighton Radiology Education Server Home Page: http://medicine.creighton.edu/radiology/main.html
The Web page of the Creighton University Division of Radiology provides information not only about the department and its resources, but also links to a set of review notes that will be of interest to both residents and practicing radiologists. This comprehensive set of notes would be of great utility to those contemplating the written or oral boards.

University of Alabama at Birmingham: http://www.rad.uab.edu
This Web site provides information about the department of radiology at the University of Birmingham, but also provides impressive links to hundreds of teaching cases. Additionally, there is information about residency programs and fellowships as well as newsletters and general information.

A
A.I. Dupont Children's Hospital, Medical Imaging:
   http://www.nemours.org/no/de/aidhc/svcs/medical_imaging.html

Alabama
University of Alabama at Birmingham Home Page: *http://main.uab.edu/*
Albert Einstein Medical Center: *http://www.einstein.edu/hp/res_diag_rad.html*

Arizona

University of Arizona, Department of Radiology:
http://www.radioalogy.arizona.edu/

B

Baylor Radiology: *http://www.bcm.tmc.edu/radiology/*
Beth Israel Hospital Department of Radiology:
http://www.bih.harvard.edu/radiology/
Boston University Medical Center Department of Radiology:
http://www.bumc.bu.edu/Departments/HomeMain.asp?DepartmentID=73
Bowman Gray School of Medicine: Division of Radiologic Sciences:
http://www.rad.bgsm.edu
Bridgeport Hospital:
http://www.bridgeporthospital.org/gme/residency/radiology/index.html
BrighamRAD, Department of Radiology, Brigham and Women's Hospital:
http://brighamrad.harvard.edu/
Brown University: *http://www.brown.edu/Departments/Diagnostic_Imaging*

C

California

Ceders-Sinai Medical Center Department of Radiology:
http://www.csmc.edu/imaging/
Ceders-Sinai Medical Center, Nuclear Medicine: *http://www.csmc.edu/imaging/*
Loma Linda School of Medicine, Radiology and Surgery:
http://www.llu.edu/llumc/radiology/
Stanford University Radiology Department: *http://www-radiology.stanford.edu/*
University of California Davis, Home Page:
http://www.ucdavis.edu/index.shtml
University of California L.A., Department of Radiological Sciences:
http://www.radsci.ucla.edu/
University of California San Diego, Department of Radiology:
http://medicine.ucsd.edu/radiology/
University of California San Francisco, Department of Radiology:
http://www.radiology.ucsf.edu/
U.C.S.F. Ultrasound Department: *http://ultrasound.ucsf.edu/*
University of Southern California, Department of Radiology:
http://www.usc.edu/schools/medicine/academic_departments/radiology/index.html
Cardiovascular and Interventional Radiology, University of Minnesota:
http://www.med.umn.edu/radiology/cvrad/
Case Western Reserve University: *http://www.uhrad.com/Default.htm*
Children's Hospital Boston, Department of Radiology:
http://www.childrenshospital.org/radiology/
Children's Hospital Boston, Nuclear Medicine:
http://nucmedweb.tch.harvard.edu/

Children's Hospital Medical Center Cincinnati, Department of Radiology:
  http://www.cincinnatichildrens.org/Services/Departments-Divisions/
  Radiology_and_Medical_Imaging/default.htm
Children's Mercy Hospital, Radiology: *http://www.childrens-mercy.org/*
  MSO/dept/default.asp

Colorado
University of Colorado Health Science Center, Radiology:
  http://www.uchsc.edu/uh/radiology/
Columbia Presbyterian Medical Center, Radiology Department:
  http://cpmcnet.columbia.edu/dept/radiology/

Connecticut
Yale University Department of Diagnostic Radiology: *http://130.132.234.113/*
Cornell Medical Center, Department of Radiology:
  http://www.nycornell.org/radiology/_&
  http://www.nycornell.org/radiology/residencies.html
Creighton Radiology Education Server Home Page:
  http://medicine.creighton.edu/radiology/index.html

D

Delaware
A.I. Dupont Children's Hospital, Medical Imaging:
  http://www.nemours.org/no/de/aidhc/svcs/medical_imaging.html
Department of Academic Radiology, University of Nottingham:
  http://www.nottingham.ac.uk/radiology/
Department of Biomedical Science, Anglia Polytechnic University:
  http://www.apu.ac.uk/appsci/lifesci/lifepath/biological_sciences.htm
Department of Diagnostic Imaging—Rhode Island Hospital, Brown University:
  http://www.brown.edu/Departments/Diagnostic_Imaging/
Department of Diagnostic Radiology, Cukurova University:
  http://lokman.cu.edu.tr/radiology/
Department of Diagnostic Radiology, Dalhousie University:
  http://www.medicine.dal.ca/home/deptadmin/clinical.htm
Department of Diagnostic Radiology, McGill University:
  http://www.rad.mgh.mcgill.ca/
Department of Diagnostic Radiology, Queen Mary Hospital, Hong Kong:
  http://www.ha.org.hk/qmh/rd/drdhome.htm
Department of Diagnostic Radiology, University of Kentucky:
  http://www.mc.uky.edu/medicine/radiology.asp
Department of Diagnostic Radiology, University of Marburg:
  http://www.med.uni-marburg.de/mzrad.html

Department of Diagnostic Radiology, University of Maryland Medicine:
http://www.umm.edu/diagnosticrad/
Department of Diagnostic Radiology, University of Turku:
http://www.utu.fi/med/radiology/
Department of Diagnostic Radiology, University of Wales:
http://www.uwcm.ac.uk/uwcm/dr/
Department of Diagnostic Radiology, Wayne State University/Detroit Medical
Center: *http://www.med.wayne.edu/diagRadiology/wsuhomepage.html*
Department of Diagnostic Radiology, Yale University:
http://info.med.yale.edu/diagrad/
Department of Diagnostic Radiology and Nuclear Medicine, Rush-
Presbyterian-St. Luke's Medical Center: *http://www.rad.rpslmc.edu/out.html*
Department of Diagnostic Radiology and Organ Imaging, Prince of Wales
Hospital: *http://www.ha.org.hk:80/pwh/special/radio01.html*
Department of Diagnostic Radiology and Nuclear Medicine, University of
Western Ontario: *http://radnuc.ihsc.on.ca/uwo/*
Department of Experimental Radiology, Erasmus University Rotterdam:
http://www.eur.nl/FGG/RDIAG/
Department of Imaging, Cedars-Sinai Medical Center:
http://www.csmc.edu/imaging/
Department of Medical Imaging, duPont Hospital for Children 1:
http://www.nemours.org/no/de/aidhc/svcs/medical_imaging.html
Department of Medical Imaging, duPont Hospital for Children 2:
http://gait.aidi.udel.edu/res695/homepage/pd_ortho/xray/xrayhp.htm
Department of Medical Imaging, Canberra Hospital:
http://www.canberrahospital.act.gov.au/specialist/medical_imaging/imaging.htm
Department of Medical Imaging, University of Toronto:
http://www.utoronto.ca/imaging/
Department of Medical Physics, University of Wisconsin:
http://www.medphysics.wisc.edu/
Department of NMR Spectroscopy, Bijvoet Center for Biomolecular Research:
http://www-nmr.chem.uu.nl/
Department of Nuclear Engineering, Univiersity of California, Berkeley:
http://www.nuc.berkeley.edu/
Department of Nuclear Medicine, Albert Szent-Gy Medical University:
http://ss10.numed.szote.u-szeged.hu
Department of Nuclear Medicine, Hokkaido University:
http://soi.med.hokudai.ac.jp/clinical-e.html
Department of Nuclear Medicine, Kanazawa University:
http://web.kanazawa-u.ac.jp/~med23/
Department of Nuclear Medicine, Physics Group, University of Massachusetts
Medical Center:
*http://www.umassmed.edu/externalwindow.cfm?URL=http://wachusett.umass
med.edu/&Link=http://www.umassmed.edu/nuclear_med/&DeptName=
Nuclear%20Medicine*

Department of Nuclear Medicine, St. Vincent's Hospital and Medical Center:
http://www.nucmedicine.com/

Department of Nuclear Medicine, State University of New York (SUNY),
Buffalo: *http://www.nucmed.buffalo.edu/*

Department of Nuclear Medicine, University of Massachusetts:
http://www.umassmed.edu/nuclear_med/

Department of Nuclear Medicine and Diagnostic Imaging, Kyoto University:
http://www-dnm.kuhp.kyoto-u.ac.jp/index-e.html

Department of Nuclear Medicine Physics, Cedars-Sinai Medical Center:
http://www.csmc.edu/medphys/nucmed/default.html

Departments of Pediatric Imaging and Pathology, Children's Hospital,
Birmingham: *http://WWW.UAB.EDU/pedradpath/*

Department of Pediatric Radiology, Women and Children's Hospital Vall
d'Hebron: *http://www.vhebron.es/vhang.htm*

Department of Physics, Lund University: *http://www.fysik.lu.se/*

Department of Physics, McGill University: *http://www.physics.mcgill.ca/*

Department of Physics, University of Texas, Southwestern:
http://www.rad.swmed.edu/PhysWeb/

Department of Radiologic Sciences, Medical College of Georgia:
http://www.mcg.edu/sah/radsci/

Department of Radiological Sciences, University of California, Los Angeles:
http://www.radsci.ucla.edu/

Department of Radiology, Baylor College of Medicine:
http://www.bcm.tmc.edu/radiology/

Department of Radiology, Beth Israel Deaconess:
http://www.bih.harvard.edu/radiology/ &
http://radiology.bidmc.harvard.edu/

Department of Radiology, Boston University:
http://www.bumc.bu.edu/Departments/HomeMain.asp?
DepartmentID=73

Department of Radiology, Case Western Reserve University:
http://www.uhrad.com/

Department of Radiology, Children's Hospital Vall d'Hebron:
http://www.vhebron.es/vhang.htm

Department of Radiology, Children's Hospital, Boston:
http://web1.tch.harvard.edu/radiology/

Department of Radiology, Columbia-Presbyterian Medical Center:
http://cpmcnet.columbia.edu/dept/radiology/

Department of Radiology, Cornell Medical Center, New York Hospital:
http://www.nycornell.org/radiology/

Department of Radiology, Cukurova University: *http://med.cu.edu.tr/radiology/*

Department of Radiology, Dartmouth-Hitchcock Medical Center:
http://www.hitchcock.org/webpage.cfm?org_id=72

Department of Radiology, Duke University: *http://www.radweb.mc.duke.edu*

Department of Radiology, Emory University:
http://www.emory.edu/RADIOLOGY/
Department of Radiology, George Washington University:
http://www.gwumc.edu/edu/radiology/open.htm
Department of Radiology, Georgetown University:
http://www.dml.georgetown.edu/depts/radiology/
Department of Radiology, Harvard Medical School:
http://www.hmcnet.harvard.edu/radiology/radiology.html
Department of Radiology, Hospital Materno-Infantil Vall d'Hebron:
http://www.xtec.es/escola/esc_hosp/mhebro/
Department of Radiology, Indiana University:
http://www.indyrad.iupui.edu/homepage.htm
Department of Radiology, Kokkaido University:
http://radi.med.hokudai.ac.jp/index.html
Department of Radiology, Long Island Jewish Medical Center:
http://www.lij.edu/lijh/radiology/radiology.html
Department of Radiology, Madigan Army Medical Center:
http://www.mamc.amedd.army.mil/mamc/depts.htm
Department of Radiology, Mahidol University:
http://www.mahidol.ac.th/mahidol/si/radio.html
Department of Radiology, McMaster University:
http://www-fhs.mcmaster.ca/radiology/
Department of Radiology, Medical College of Virginia:
http://www.radiology.vcu.edu/
Department of Radiology, Medical College of Wisconsin:
http://www.mcw.edu/radiology/
Department of Radiology, Memorial Sloan-Kettering Cancer Center:
http://www.mskcc.org/mskcc/html/44.cfm
Department of Radiology, MetroHealth Medical Center:
http://www.metrohealth.org/clinical/radiology/
Department of Radiology, Miami Children's Hospital:
http://www.mch.com/clinical/radiology/index.html
Department of Radiology, Michigan State University:
http://haven.rad.msu.edu/
Department of Radiology, Mount Sinai School of Medicine:
http://www.mssm.edu/radiology/home-page.html
Department of Radiology, Nagasaki University Hospital:
http://www.med.nagasaki-u.ac.jp/radiology/case1.html
Department of Radiology, New York University:
http://radnyu.med.nyu.edu/index.html
Department of Radiology, Oregon Health Sciences University:
http://www.ohsu.edu/ps-DiagRadiol/index.html
Department of Radiology, PennState Geisinger Medical Center:
http://www.geisinger.org/services/radiology/radiology_index.shtml

Department of Radiology, Pennsylvania State University:
  http://www.rad.upenn.edu/Dept.html
Department of Radiology, Robert Wood Johnson Medical School: *http://rwj-rad.rwjuh.edu/*
Department of Radiology, St. Bartholomew's and the Royal London School of
  Medicine and Dentistry of Queen Mary and Westfield College, University
  of London: *http://www.mds.qmw.ac.uk/radiol/*
Department of Radiology, St. Paul's Hospital:
  http://wwwrad.pulmonary.ubc.ca/StPaulsRadiol.html
Department of Radiology, Stanford University:
  http://www-radiology.stanford.edu/
Department of Radiology, State University of New York, Brooklyn:
  http://radiology.hscbklyn.edu/
Department of Radiology, State University of New York, Stony Brook:
  http://www.uhmc.sunysb.edu:8080/
Department of Radiology, State University of New York, Syracuse:
  http://www.upstate.edu/cancer/cardio.shtml
Department of Radiology, Thomas Jefferson University:
  http://www.jeffersonhospital.org/radiology/
Department of Radiology, Tokushima University Hospital:
  http://www.med.tokushima-u.ac.jp/hospital/
Department of Radiology, Tulane University:
  http://www.mcl.tulane.edu/departments/Radiology/rad_home.htm
Department of Radiology, University of Alabama, Birmingham:
  http://www.rad.uab.edu
Department of Radiology, University of Alberta:
  http://www.ualberta.ca/~raddi/
Department of Radiology, University of Arizona:
  http://www.radiology.arizona.edu/
Department of Radiology, University of Athens: *http://www.rad.uoa.gr/*
Department of Radiology, University of British Columbia:
  http://www1.stpaulshosp.bc.ca
Department of Radiology, University of California, Davis:
  http://www-radiology.ucdmc.ucdavis.edu/
Department of Radiology, University of California, San Francisco:
  http://www.radiology.ucsf.edu/
Department of Radiology, University of Cambridge:
  http://www.medschl.cam.ac.uk/rad/radiol.html
Department of Radiology, University of Chicago:
  http://www-radiology.uchicago.edu
Department of Radiology, University of Cincinnati:
  http://www.med.uc.edu/departme/radiol/
Department of Radiology, University of Colorado:
  http://www.uchsc.edu/uh/radiology/
Department of Radiology, University of Florida: *http://www.xray.ufl.edu/*

Department of Radiology, University of Iowa:
http://www.radiology.uiowa.edu/
Department of Radiology, University of Kansas: *http://www.rad.kumc.edu/*
Department of Radiology, University of Manitoba:
http://www.umanitoba.ca/faculties/medicine/radiology/hsc/index.html
Department of Radiology, University of Marburg: *http://www.med.uni-marburg.de/mzrad.html*
Department of Radiology, University of Massachusetts:
http://www.umassmed.edu/radiology/
Department of Radiology, University of Melbourne:
http://www.radiology.unimelb.edu.au/
Department of Radiology, University of Miami:
http://www.miami.edu/UMH/CDA/UMH_Main/1.1770.2576-1.00.html
Department of Radiology, University of Michigan:
http://www.rad.med.umich.edu/
Department of Radiology, University of Minnesota:
http://www.med.umn.edu/radiology
Department of Radiology, University of Mississippi: *http://rad.umc.edu/*
Department of Radiology, University of North Carolina, Chapel Hill:
http://www.med.unc.edu/radiology/
Department of Radiology, University of Pennsylvania:
http://www.rad.upenn.edu/
Department of Radiology, University of Pisa:
http://www.rad.unipi.it.pagina_rad.html
Department of Radiology, University of Rochester:
http://www.urmc.rochester.edu/smd/rad/
Department of Radiology, University of Sydney:
http://www.usyd.edu.au/su/radiology/usindex.htm
Department of Radiology, University of Tennessee, Knoxville:
http://www.utmedicalcenter.org/radiology/
Department of Radiology, University of Tennessee, Memphis:
http://www.utmem.edu/radiology/
Department of Radiology, University of Texas, Houston:
http://www.uth.tmc.edu/radiology/
Department of Radiology, University of Texas, Southwestern:
http://www.rad.swmed.edu/
Department of Radiology, University of Texas Health Science Center, San
Antonio: *http://radiology.uthscsa.edu/*
Department of Radiology, University of Utah: *http://amber.med.utah.edu*
Department of Radiology, University of Virginia:
http://hsc.virginia.edu/medicine/clinical/radiology/home.html
Department of Radiology, University of Washington:
http://www.rad.washington.edu:80/
Department of Radiology, Vancouver Hospital:
http://web.ucs.ubc.ca/aldrich/home.htm

Department of Radiology, Vanderbilt University:
  http://www.mc.Vanderbilt.Edu/radiology/
Department of Radiology, Virginia Commonwealth University:
  http://www.radiology.vcu.edu/index.htm
Department of Radiology, Virginia Mason Medical Center:
  http://www.vmmc.org/dbGraduateMedicalEducation/sec68332.htm
Department of Radiology, Virtual Hospital:
  http://www.vh.org/Patients/IHB/Radiology.html
Department of Radiology, Walter Reed Army Medical Center:
  http://www.wramc.amedd.army.mil/departments/wramcrad
Department of Radiology, Wayne State University/Detroit Medical Center:
  http://www.med.wayne.edu/diagRadiology/
Department of Radiology, Weill Medical College of Cornell University:
  http://www.nycornell.org/radiology/
Department of Radiology, Westmead Hospital:
  http://www.usyd.edu.au/su/radiology/oldindex.html
Department of Radiology and Nuclear Medicine, Thomas Jefferson University
  Hospital: *http://www.jeffersonhospital.org/radiology/e3front.dll?durki=3890*
Department of Radiology and Nuclear Medicine, Uniformed Service
  University of the Health Sciences:
  http://radlinux1.usuf1.usuhs.mil/rad/mainpage.html
Department of Radiology and Radiological Sciences, Vanderbilt University:
  http://www.mc.vanderbilt.edu/vumcdept/radio.html
Department of Radiotherapy and Oncology, Queen Mary Hospital:
  http://www.ha.org.hk/qmh/rt/
Department of Radiotherapy, University Hospital of Ghent:
  http://krtkg1.rug.ac.be
Division of Diagnostic and Interventional Radiology, University of Pisa:
  http://www.rad.unipi.it
Division of Diagnostic Imaging, University of Texas—M.D. Anderson:
  http://www.mdanderson.org/departments/radiology/
Division of Functional Diagnostic Imaging Biomedical Research Center,
  Osaka University: *http://www.med.osaka-u.ac.jp/pub/general*
Division of Image Science and Technology, University of Kansas:
  http://www.kumc.edu/dist/
Division of Magnetic Resonance Research, Johns Hopkins University:
  http://www.mri.jhu.edu/div_mri_res/
Division of Neuroradiology, University of Cincinnati:
  http://www.med.uc.edu/departme/radiol/neurorad/neurorad.htm
Division of Nuclear Medicine, Cedars-Sinai Medical Center:
  http://www.csmc.edu/imaging/
Division of Nuclear Medicine, Children's Hospital, Boston:
  http://nucmedweb.tch.harvard.edu/
Division of Nuclear Medicine, Department of Radiology, New York
  University: *http://radnyu.med.nyu.edu/index.html*

Division of Nuclear Medicine, Mallinckrodt Institute of Radiology:
  http://gamma.wustl.edu/
Division of Nuclear Medicine, Siriraj Hospital:
  http://www.mahidol.ac.th/mahidol/si/nmst.html
Division of Nuclear Medicine, St. Louis University: *http://gamma.wustl.edu/*
Division of Nuclear Medicine, University of Arizona:
  http://www.medicine.arizona.edu/depts/radiology.html
Division of Nuclear Medicine, University of British Columbia:
  http://www.ubc.ca/academic/fac_schools.html#medicine
Division of Nuclear Medicine, University of Kansas:
  http://www.rad.kumc.edu/users/jtraylor/nucmed/index.htm
Division of Nuclear Medicine, University of Utah:
  http://www.uuhsc.med.utah.edu/rad/nucmed/nuchome.html
Division of Oral and Maxillofacial Radiology, Dalhousie University:
  http://bpass.dentistry.dal.ca/
Division of Physiologic Imaging, University of Iowa:
  http://everest.radiology.uiowa.edu:80/home.html
Division of Radiation Oncology, Arthur G. James Cancer Hospital and
  Research Institute: *http://www-radonc.med.ohio-state.edu/*
Division of Radiologic Sciences, Bowman Gray School of Medicine, Wake
  Forest University: *http://www.rad.bgsm.edu/*
Division of Radiological Sciences, United Medical and Dental Schools of
  Guy's and St. Thomas' Hospitals:
  http://www.kcl.ac.uk/depsta/medicine/rsme/index.html
Duke University Radiology Department: *http://www.radweb.mc.duke.edu/*

E
Eastern Virginia Medical School: *http://www.evms.edu/radiology/indx.html*
Emory University Radiology Home Page:
  http://www.emory.edu/RADIOLOGY/index.html &
  http://www.emory.edu/RADIOLOGY/resident.html

F

Florida
University of Florida Department of Radiology: *http://www.xray.ufl.edu/*
University of Miami School of Medicine Radiology Department:
  http://www.miami.edu/UMH/CDA/UMH_Main/1.1770.2576-1.00.html

G
George Washington University Department of Radiology:
  http://www.gwumc.edu/edu/radiology &
  http://www.gwumc.edu/edu/radiology/index.htm
Georgetown University Department of Radiology:
  http://www.dml.georgetown.edu/depts/radiology/

Georgia

Emory University Radiology Home Page:
http://www.emory.edu/RADIOLOGY/index.html
Medical College of Georgia Dept. of Radiology:
http://www.radiology.mcg.edu/
Graduate Hospital, Philadelphia:
http://www.graduatehospital.com/graduatehospital/default.asp

H

Harvard-Beth Israel Hospital: *http://radiology.bidmc.harvard.edu/*
Harvard-Brigham and Women's Hospital:
http://www.brighamandwomens.org/radiology/

I

Illinois

Loyola, Section of Nuclear Medicine—LUNIS Public Home Page:
http://lunis.luc.edu/lunis
Northwestern University Department of Radiology:
http://www.radiology.northwestern.edu/
Rush Presbyterian St. Lukes Department of Radiology:
http://www.rush.edu/patients/radoncology/index.html
University of Chicago Radiology Home Page:
http://www.radiology.uchicago.edu/

Indiana

Indiana University Radiology: *http://www.indyrad.iupui.edu/homepage.htm* &
http://www.indyrad.iupui.edu/misc/residency.html

Iowa

University of Iowa, Department of Radiology:
http://www.radiology.uiowa.edu/

J

Johns Hopkins Department of Radiology:
http://www.hopkinsmedicine.org/departments.html

K

Kansas

University of Kansas Medical Center Radiology Home Page:
http://www3.kumc.edu/radiology/
University of Kansas Medical Center—Nuclear Medicine Department:
http://www.rad.kumc.edu/nucmed/

Kentucky

University of Kentucky College of Medicine: Diagnostic Radiology
Department: *http://www.mc.uky.edu/medicine/radiology.asp*

L

Loma Linda School of Medicine, Radiology and Surgery:
http://www.llu.edu/llumc/radiology/
Long Island Jewish Med. Center Department of Radiology:
http://www.lij.edu/lijh/radiology/radiology.html &
http://www.lij.edu/lijh/radiology/training.html

Louisiana

Tulane University Department of Radiology:
http://www1.omi.tulane.edu/departments/radiology/rad_home.htm
Loyola, Section of Nuclear Medicine—LUNIS Public Home Page:
http://lunis.luc.edu/lunis/

M

Madigan Army Medical Center Department of Radiology:
http://www.mamc.amedd.army.mil/mamc/depts.htm
Magnetic Resonance Department, University Hospital Gent in Belgium:
http://mri2-gw00.rug.ac.be/
Mallinckrodt Institute of Radiology: *http://www.mir.wustl.edu/*

Maryland

Johns Hopkins Department of Radiology:
http://www.hopkinsmedicine.org/departments.html
Uniformed Services University of Health Sciences: Radiology on the Web:
http://rad.usuhs.mil/index.html
University of Maryland Department of Diagnostic Radiology:
http://www.umm.edu/diagnosticrad/

Massachusetts

Beth Israel Hospital Department of Radiology:
http://radiology.bidmc.harvard.edu/
Boston University Medical Center Department of Radiology:
http://www.bumc.bu.edu/departments/homemain.asp?departmentid=73
Boston VAMC Radiology: *http://www.gentili.net/TF98/29.htm*
BrigamRad, Brigham and Women's Hospital, Harvard Children's Hospital
Boston, Department of Radiology: *http://brighamrad.harvard.edu/*
Children's Hospital Boston, Nuclear Medicine:
http://www.childrenshospital.org/cfapps/CHprogDisplay.cfm?Dept=
Radiology&Prog=Nuclear%20Medicine
Massachusetts General Hospital: *http://www.mgh.harvard.edu/*

University of Massachusetts Medical Center Department of Nuclear Medicine:
http://www.umassmed.edu/nuclear_med/
McGaw Medical Center of NWU: *http://www.nums.nwu.edu/gme/diaradio.htm*
McMaster University: *http://www-fhs.mcmaster.ca/radiology/*
MDA—M.D. Anderson, Division of Diagnostic Imaging:
http://rpiwww.mdacc.tmc.edu/di/
Medical College of Georgia Department of Radiology:
http://www.radiology.mcg.edu/
Medical College of Pennsylvania Radiology Web Page:
http://www.drexel.edu/med/radiology/
Medical College of Virginia at VCU:
http://www.radiology.vcu.edu/residency.htm
Medical College of Wisconsin Department of Radiology:
http://www.mcw.edu/radiology
Medical Physics, Medical College of Wisconsin:
http://www.mcw.edu/medphys/
Medical Physics, University of Aberdeen: *http://www.biomed.abdn.ac.uk/*
Memorial Sloan-Kettering Department of Radiology:
http://www.mskcc.org/mskcc/html/56.cfm_Michigan
Michigan State University Radiology: *http://www.rad.msu.edu/*
University of Michigan Radiology Home Page: *http://www.rad.med.umich.edu/*
Wayne State University Detroit Medical Center: Diagnostic Radiology:
http://www.med.wayne.edu/diagradiology/wsuhomepage.html

Minnesota
Mayo Clinic Department of Radiology: *http://www.mayo.edu/mcr/*
University of Minnesota, Department of Radiology:
http://www.med.umn.edu/radiology/index.html
University of Minnesota Pediatric Imaging Section:
http://www.tc.umn.edu/~hitex001/pedsimage/peds.html

Mississippi
UMC Department of Radiology: *http://rad.umc.edu/*

Missouri
Children's Mercy Hospital, Radiology: *http://www.childrens-mercy-org/*
MSO/dept/default.asp
Mallinckrodt Institute of Radiology: *http://www.mir.wustl.edu/*
Mount Sinai School of Medicine: Radiology:
http://www.mssm.edu/radiology/home-page.html
MRI Education Foundation: *http://64.49.193.202/*

N
Nagasaki Department of Radiology: *http://www.med.nagasaki-u.ac.jp/radiology/case1.html*

Nebraska

New York
Columbia Presbyterian Medical Center, Radiology Department:
http://cpmcnet.columbia.edu/dept/radiology/
Cornell Medical Center, Department of Radiology:
http://www.nycornell.org/radiology/
Long Island Jewish Medical Center Department of Radiology:
http://www.lij.edu/lijh/radiology/radiology.html
Mount Sinai School of Medicine: Radiology:
http://www.mssm.edu/radiology/home-page.html
NYU Medical School Department of Radiology:
http://radnyu.med.nyu.edu/index.html
Memorial Sloan-Kettering Department of Radiology:
http://www.mskcc.org/mskcc/html/56.cfm
S.U.N.Y.: Stony Brook, Department of Radiology:
http://www.uhmc.sunysb.edu:8080/
University of Rochester Medical Center, Department of Radiology:
http://www.urmc.rochester.edu/smd/rad/

New Jersey
Robert Wood Johnson Medical School Department of Radiology:
http://rwjms.umdnj.edu/departments/

North Carolina
Bowman Gray School of Medicine: Division of Radiologic Sciences:
http://www.rad.bgsm.edu/
Duke University Radiology Department: *http://www.radweb.mc.duke.edu/*
University of North Carolina Radiology Website:
http://www.med.unc.edu/depts_radiology.htm
North Shore University Radiology Home Page:
http://www.northshorelij.com/visit/index.cfm
NYU Medical School Department of Radiology:
http://radnyu.med.nyu.edu/index.html

O

Ohio
Children's Hospital Medical Center Cincinnati, Department of Radiology:
http://www.cincinnatichildrens.org/services/departments-divisions/radiology_and_medical_imaging/default.htm

University of Cincinnati, Department of Radiology:
  http://www.med.uc.edu/departme/radiol/index.html
University of Cincinnati Division of Neuroradiology Home Page:
  http://www.med.uc.edu/departme/radiol/neurorad/neurorad.htm
University Hospitals of Cleveland and Case Western Reserve University,
  Radiology: *http://www.uhrad.com/default.htm*

Oregon
Oregon Health Sciences University, Dotter Interventional Institute:
  http://www.ohsu.edu/dotter/
Oregon Health Sciences University: *http://www.ohsu.edu/*
  ps-DiagRadiol/radres.htm

P
Pediatric Imaging Section, University of Minnesota:
  http://www.tc.umn.edu/nlhome/m122/hitex001/pedsimage/
Pediatric Radiology Section, University of Minnesota:
  http://www.tc.umn.edu/nlhome/m122/hitex001/pedsimage/peds.html
PennState Geisinger Medical Center:
  http://www.geisinger.org/services/radiology/radiology_index.shtml
Penn State Department of Radiology: *http://www.xray.hmc.psu.edu/*

Pennsylvania
Thomas Jefferson University Hospital, Radiology and Nuclear Medicine:
  http://www.jeffersonhospital.org/radiology/e3front.dll?durki=3890
University of Pennsylvania Medical Center Radiology Home Page:
  http://www.med.upenn.edu/radiology.html
University of Pittsburgh Medical Center—Radiology Department:
  http://www.radiology.upmc.edu/
Peoria Radiology Associates: *http://www.peoria-radiology.com/*

R
Radiodiagnostik Homburg: *http://www.med-rz.uni-*
  sb.de/med_fak/radiodiagnostik/index.html
Radiologie, Universitätsklinikum Benjamin Franklin: *http://www.medizin.*
  fu-berlin.de/radio/radio.html
Radiology Research Section, University of Texas Medical Branch, Galveston:
  http://radweb.utmb.edu/
Radiosurgery, University of Florida: *http://radsurg.ufl.edu/*

Rhode Island
Department of Diagnostic Imaging—Rhode Island Hospital, Brown University:
  http://www.brown.edu/Departments/Diagnostic_Imaging/
Robert Wood Johnson Medical School Department of Radiology:
  http://rwjms.umdnj.edu/departments/

Rochester General Hospital: *http://www.viahealth.org/radres/*
Rush Presbyterian St. Lukes Department of Radiology:
　http://www.rad.rpslmc.edu/_&_http://www.rad.rpslmc.edu/training.html

S

Scott and White/Texas A&: *http://www.sw.org/depts/rad/gme/rad.htm*
Section of Neuroradiology, University of Brescia:
　http://www.unibs.it/~gasparo/neuro.html
Section of Neuroradiology, University of California San Francisco:
　http://www.neurorad.ucsf.edu/
Section of Nuclear Medicine, Kapiolani Medical Center for Women and
　Children: *http://www.kapionlani.org/facilities/children.html*
Section of Nuclear Medicine, Loyola University: *http://www.lunis.luc.edu/*
Section of Nuclear Medicine, University of Illinois:
　http://www.uic.edu/com/uhrd/nucmed/homepage.htm
Section of Pediatric Radiology, Stanford University:
　http://pichon.stanford.edu/clinical/peds.html
Section of Pediatric Radiology, University of Chicago:
　http://www-radiology.uchicago.edu/sections/pediatric.html
Section of Pediatric Radiology, University of Manitoba:
　http://www.umanitoba.ca:80/faculties/medicine/radiology/hsc/prad.html
Section of Radiation Oncology, West Virginia University:
　http://www.hsc.wvu.edu/radrx/
Section of Radiological Sciences, University of Torino: *http://www.unito.it/*
Sez.Scienze Radiologiche, University of Modena:
　http://imoax1.unimo.it/~radmo/welcome.html
St. Luke's-Roosevelt (DOCNET)—Department of Radiology:
　http://www.wehealnewyork.org/professionals/residency/slr_radiology.html
Stanford University Radiology Department: *http://www-radiology.stanford.edu/*
　& *http://www-radiology.stanford.edu/education/Residency.html*
SUNY: Brooklyn, Department of Radiology:
　http://www.hscbklyn.edu/uhbclinics/RADIOLOGY.html
SUNY: Stony Brook, Department of Radiology:
　http://www.informatics.sunysb.edu/radiology/
SUNY: Syracuse, Radiology Department Home Page:
　http://www.upstate.edu/radiology/residency.htm

T

Tennessee
University of Tennessee Medical Center at Knoxville:
　http://www.utmedicalcenter.org/homeie455plus.htm
Vanderbilt University Medical Center, Department of Radiology and
　Radiological Sciences: *http://www.mc.vanderbilt.edu/radiology/*

Texas

Baylor Radiology Home Page: *http://www.bcm.tmc.edu/radiology/*

MDA—M.D. Anderson, Division of Diagnostic Imaging:
http://www.mdanderson.org/departments/radiology/

University of Texas Medical School, Houston—Department of Radiology:
http://www.uth.tmc.edu/radiology/

University of Texas Southwestern Radiology Department:
http://www.rad.swmed.edu/

Wilford Hall Medical Center, Lackland AFB: *http://www.whmc.af.mil/*

Thomas Jefferson University Hospital, Radiology and Nuclear Med:
http://www.rad.tju.edu/education/residencies.html &
http://www.jeffersonhospital.org/radiology/e3front.dll?durki=3890

Tulane University Department of Radiology:
http://www.mcl.tulane.edu/departments/Radiology/rad_home.htm

U

Uniformed Services University of Health Sciences:
http://radlinux1.usuf1.usuhs.mil/rad/

University of Alabama-Birmingham: *http://www.rad.uab.edu*

University of Arizona, Department of Radiology:
http://www.radiology.arizona.edu/

University of British Columbia: *http://www1.stpaulshosp.bc.ca/*

University of California Davis, Home Page:
http://www-radiology.ucdmc.ucdavis.edu/

University of California Irvine, Radiological Sciences:
http://www.ucihs.uci.edu/radonc/

University of California Los Angeles, Department of Radiological Sciences:
http://www.radsci.ucla.edu/

University of California San Diego, Department of Radiology:
http://medicine.ucsd.edu/Radiology/

University of California San Francisco, Department of Radiology:
http://radiology.ucsf.edu/

University of California San Francisco Ultrasound Department:
http://ultrasound.ucsf.edu/

University of Chicago Radiology: *http://www-radiology.uchicago.edu/*

University of Cincinnati, Department of Radiology:
http://www.med.uc.edu/departme/radiol/

University of Cincinnati Division of Neuroradiology Home Page:
http://www.med.uc.edu/departme/radiol/neurorad/neurorad.htm

Univ. of Colorado Health Science Center, Radiology:
http://www.uchsc.edu/uh/radiology/

University of Florida Department of Radiology: *http://www.xray.ufl.edu/*

University Hospitals of Cleveland and Case Western Reserve University,
Radiology: *http://www.uhrad.com/*

University of Iowa Department of Radiology: *http://www.radiology.uiowa.edu/*
University of Kansas Medical Center Radiology Home Page:
   http://www.rad.kumc.edu/
University of Kansas Medical Center—Nuclear Medicine Department:
   http://www.rad.kumc.edu/nucmed/
University of Kentucky College of Medicine: Diagnostic Radiology
   Department: *http://www.mc.uky.edu/medicine/radiology.asp*
University of Maryland Department of Diagnostic Radiology:
   http://www.umm.edu/diagnosticrad/
University of Massachusetts Medical Center Department of Nuclear Medicine:
   http://www.umassmed.edu/nuclear_med/
University of Miami School of Medicine Radiology Department:
   http://www.miami.edu/UMH/CDA/UMH_Main/1.1770.2576-1.00.html
University of Michigan Radiology Home Page: *http://www.rad.med.umich.edu/*
University of Minnesota, Department of Radiology:
   http://www.med.umn.edu/radiology/
University of Minnesota Pediatric Imaging Section:
   http://www.tc.umn.edu/nlhome/m122/hitex001/pedsimage/peds.html
UMC Department of Radiology: *http://rad.umc.edu/*
University of North Carolina Radiology: *http://sunsite.unc.edu/jksmith/*
   UNC-Radiology-Webserver/mainmenu.html
University of Pennsylvania Medical Center Radiology Home Page:
   http://www.rad.upenn.edu/
University of Pittsburgh Medical Center—Radiology Department:
   http://www.radiology.upmc.edu/
University of Rochester Medical Center, Department of Radiology:
   http://www.urmc.rochester.edu/smd/Rad/;
   http://www.urmc.rochester.edu/SMD/Rad/Radhome.html
University of Southern California, Department of Radiology:
   http://www.usc.edu/schools/medicine/academic_departments/radiology/
University of Tennessee Medical Center at Knoxville:
   http://www.utmedicalcenter.org/homeie455plus.htm
University of Tennessee, Memphis: Department of Radiology:
   http://www.utmem.edu/radiology/
University of Texas Medical School, Houston—Department of Radiology:
   http://www.uth.tmc.edu/radiology/
University of Texas Southwestern Radiology Department:
   http://physicsgate.swmed.edu/
University of Toronto: *http://www.utoronto.ca/imaging/fellowships/intro.htm*
University of Utah, Department of Radiology: *http://www.uuhsc.utah.edu/rad/*
UVA Health Sciences Center Radiology Department:
   http://hsc.virginia.edu/medicine/clinical/radiology/educ-opps/
   residency-program.html
University of Washington Webserver: *http://www.rad.washington.edu/*
University of Western Ontario: *http://radnuc.lhsc.on.ca/uwo/*

Utah
University of Utah, Department of Radiology: *http://www.uuhsc.utah.edu/rad/*

V
Vanderbilt University Medical Center, Department of Radiology and
Radiological Sciences: *http://www.mc.vanderbilt.edu/vumcdept/radio.html*

Virginia
UVA Health Sciences Center Radiology Department:
*http://hsc.virginia.edu/medicine/clinical/radiology/educ-opps/residency-
program.html*
Virginia Mason Medical Center Department of Radiology:
http://www.vmmc.org/dbGraduateMedicalEducation/sec68332.htm

W
Walter Reed Army Medical Center Department of Radiology:
http://www.wramc.amedd.army.mil/departments/WRAMCRad/index.htm
Walter Reed NuclearMedicine Home Page:
http://www.wramc.amedd.army.mil/departments/nuclear/

Washington
University of Washington Webserver: *http://www.rad.washington.edu/*
Virginia Mason Medical Center Department of Radiology:
http://www.virginiamason.org/dbradiology/default.htm

Washington D.C.
George Washington University Department of Radiology:
http://www.gwumc.edu/edu/radiology/open.htm
Georgetown University Department of Radiology:
http://www.georgetown.edu/departments/radiology/
Walter Reed Army Medical Center Department of Radiology:
http://www.wramc.amedd.army.mil/
Walter Reed Nuclear Medicine Home Page:
http://www.wramc.amedd.army.mil/departments/nuclear
Washington University—MIR: *http://www.mir.wustl.edu/mir.html*
Wayne State University/Detroit Medical Center: Diagnostic Radiology:
http://www.med.wayne.edu/diagRadiology/wsuhomepage.html
Wilford Hall Medical Lackland AFB: *http://www.whmc.af.mil/*

Wisconsin
Medical College of Wisconsin Department of Radiology:
http://www.mcw.edu/radiology/

Y

Yale University Department of Diagnostic Radiology:
http://info.med.yale.edu/diagrad/_&
http://info.med.yale.edu/diagrad/rf_info.html

Z

Zentrum der Radiologie, Klinikum der Johann Wolfgang Goethe—
Universität/ZRAD: *http://141.2.61.48/zrad.htm*

Vendors

AGFA Medical: http://www.agfa.com/healthcare/us/
The AGFA Web site provides links and information to the popular medical imaging vendor both in the film and PCAS circles. There is information about PACS installations as well as links to educational material the vendor provides.

Berlex: www.berlex.com
The Berlex Web site provides links to company information as well as to product information and future research efforts.

General Electric: http://www.gemedicalsystems.com/index.html
The GE medical Web site provides a vast array of information from this ubiquitous manufacturer, ranging from hardware and software to IT solutions to education. Also present is information about services, financing, productivity solutions, and accessories.

3D-Doctor: *http://www.ablesw.com/3d-doctor/*

A

A1 Alpha Space, Inc: *http://www.a1alpha.com/*
Acuson: *http://www.acuson.com*
ADAC Labs: *http://www.adaclabs.com/*
Advanced Health Education Center: *http://www.aheconline.com/*
Advanced Magnetics, Inc: *http://www.advancedmagnetics.com*
Agfa: *http://www.agfa.com/healthcare/us/*
ALI Technologies: *http://www.alitech.com/*
American Medical Sales, Inc.: *http://www.digitalams.com*
Analogic: *http://www.analogic.com/*
Anamedic: *http://www.anamedic.com/*
Applicare Medical Imaging B.V.: *http://www.applicare.com*
Associated X-Ray Imaging: *http://www.associatedxray.com/*
ATL Ultrasound: *http://www.atl.com*

B

Berlex: *http://www.berlex.com*
Biosound Esaote: *http://www.biosound.com/*
Bracco: *http://www.bracco.com/Bracco/home.htm*
BRIT Systems: *http://www.brit.com*

C

Cejka and Company: *http://www.cejka.com/*
CHILI—Teleradiology: *http://www.chili-radiology.com/*
Ciprico: *http://www.ciprico.com/*
Clark Research and Development: *http://www.clarkrd.com*
CMC Medical Imaging Systems: *http://www.123cmc.com/*
Comdisco: *http://www.comdisco.com/default.asp*
CompuRAD: *http://www.compurad.com/*

D

DaGA, Inc.: *http://www.daga.com/*
Dejarnette: *http://www.dejarnette.com/*
Diagnostix Plus, Inc.: *http://www.diagplus.com*
Diasonics: *http://www.diasonics.com/*
Diwan Chand Satyapal Aggarwal Imaging: *http://www.dcaimaging.org*
Dome Imaging Systems: *http://www.dome.com/*
DOTmed: *http://www.dotmed.com/*
dpiX: *http://www.dpix.com/*
Dynamic Healthcare Technologies: *http://www.dht.com/*

E

Elema-Schonander: *http://www.elema-schonander.com/*
Elscint: *http://www.elscint.co.il/*
EMED: *http://www.raytheon.com/e-sys/icsd/emed/emed.htm*
Epix Medical: *http://www.epixmed.com/*

F

Fischer Imaging: *http://www.fischerimaging.com*
Fonar: *http://www.fonar.com/*
Fuji: *http://www.fujimed.com/*

G

Gammex: *http://www.gammex.com/*
Gaston Radiology: *http://www.gastonradiology.com/index.html*
GE Medical Systems: *http://www.gemedicalsystems.com/index.html*
Gilbert X-Ray: *http://www.gxr.com/*
Gordon Instruments: *http://www.gordon-instruments.com/*
GTR: *http://gtrllc.com/*

H

Hayden Image Processing Group: *http://www.perceptive.com/*
Hewlett Packard: *http://www.hp/com/*
Hitachi: *http://www.hitachi.com/*
Hologic: *http://www.hologic.com/*
Howtek: *http://www.howtek.com*
H.R. Simon and Co.: *http://www.hrsimon.com/*

I

IBM Healthcare: *http://www.ibm.com/us/*
IES: *http://www.iesmri.com*
Images-on-Call: *http://www.imagesoncall.com*
Imaging Associates, Inc.: *http://www.ImagingA.com/*
Imation: *http://www.imation.com/*
Imatron: *http://www.geimatron.com/*
Immunomedics, Inc.: *http://www.immunomedics.com/*
Imnet: *http://imnet.jst.go.jp/en/*
Imperium, Inc.: *http://www.imperiuminc.com*
Info-X Inc.: *http://www.info-x-inc.com/*
InPhact: *http://www.inphact.com/*
Insight Medical Management Systems: *http://www.InsightMed.com/*
Instrumentarium: *http://www.instrumentarium.com/*
Integrity Medical Systems, Inc.: *http://www.integritymed.com/*
ISG Technologies, Inc.: *http://www.corporate-ir.net/*
   media_files/NSD/cdsw/reports/ar97.pdf

J

JPI America: *http://www.jpiamerica.com/*

K

Kenex (Electro-Medical) Ltd.: *http://www.kenex.co.uk*
Keston Group: *http://www.keston.com/*
Kodak: *http://www.kodak.com/*
Konica Medical Corp.: *http://www.konicamedical.com*

L

Lumisys: *http://www.lumisys.com/*

M

Mallinckrodt: *http://www.mallinckrodt.com/*
MarkCare Medical Systems: *http://www.mark-solutions.com/*
Medical EquipNet:
   http://www.solumed.com/medicalequipnet.cfm?ChLng=EN&refid=0

Medical X-Ray Enterprises: *http://www.mxe.com/*
Mediface: *http://www.mediface.com*
MEDIS Medical Imaging Systems: *http://www.medis.nl/*
Medison: *http://www.medison.co.kr*
Medrad: *http://www.medrad.com*
MedSim: *http://www.medsim.com/*
MedVision: *http://www.medvision.de/*
Medweb Telemedicine: *http://www.medweb.net/*
Merge Technologies: *http://www.merge.com/*
Mirus Industries: *http://www.bioscience.org/company/mirus.htm*
MRI Accreditation Consultants: *http://members.tripod.com/mrconsultants/*

N
NEC: *http://www.nec.com*
NeoVision Corp: *http://www.radiologist.com/comm1a.htm*
Nycomed Amersham: *http://www.amershamhealth.com/*

O
OEC Medical Systems: *http://www.prnewswire.com/gh/cnoc/comp/630450.html*
OTech: *http://www.otechimg.com/*
Ozrad Radiology Resources: *http://www.ozrad.com/*

P
Pacific Northwest X-Ray Inc.: *http://www.pnwx.com/*
Philips Medical Systems: *http://www.pmsna.com/*
Picker: *http://www.picker.com/*
PictureTel: *http://www.picturetel.com/*
Polaroid: *http://www.polaroid.com/*
Precision Digital: *http://www.predig.com/*

Q
Quest International, Inc.: *http://www.questinc.com/*

R
Radfiler: *http://www.radfiler.com/*
Radiology Consultants: *http://www.radiologyconsultants.com/*
RadTrak: *http://www.radtrak.com/*
RDI: *http://www.rdi-electronics.com/*
RemoteImage, LLC: *http://www.remoteimage.com*
River Oaks Imaging and Diagnostic: *http://www.riveroaksimaging.com*
Rogers Ultrasound Imaging, Inc.: *http://www.ultrasoundsales.com/*
RSTI: *http://www.rsti-training.com/*

S
S and S X-Ray: *http://www.ssxray.com/*

Sectra-Imtec: *http://www.sectra.se/medical/index.html*
Sonus Pharmaceuticals: *http://www.sonuspharma.com/*
Sony Medical Systems:
   http://bssc.sel.sony.com/Professional/webapp/Market?m=10006
Southern Medical Engineering: *http://www.alltel.net/~sme7126/*
Sterling Diagnostic Imaging: *http://www.acvr.ucdavis.edu/sponsors/agfa.html*
StorateTek: *http://www.stortek.com*
Sun Microsystems: *http://www.sun.com/*

T
TIMS: *http://www.tims.com/*
Toshiba Medical: *http://www.toshiba.com/tams/*
Tricat Imaging Center: *http://www.tricat.com*

U
US Diagnostic: *http://www.usdl.com/profile.asp*

V
ValueMed: *http://www.valuemed.net/*
Varian: *http://www.varian.com/*
Voxel Digital Holography: *http://www.voxel.com/*
VTEL Videoconferencing: *http://www.vtel.com/*

X
XiTec: *http://www.xitec.com/*

Book Vendors/Teaching Materials

A
Accesspub Interactive: *http://www.accesspub.com/*
ACR Publications Catalog: *http://webtch.com/ACRbooks/catM-R.htm*
Appleton & Lange: *http://books.mcgraw-hillcom/medical/appleton/*

B
Blackwell Science Inc.—Home Page:
   http://www.blacksci.co/uk/usa/default.htm

C
Churchill Livingstone: *http://www.churchillmed.com/*
CRC Press: *http://www.crcpress.com/*

E
Educational Symposia, Inc: *http://www.edusymp.com/*
Elsevier Science Home Page: *http://www.elsevier.com/*

H
Harvard University Press: *http://www.hup.harvard.edu/*

L
Lippincott-Raven: *http://www.lww.com/*
Lippincott Williams & Wilkins: *http://www.lww.com/*
Little, Brown: *http://212.22.11.106/*
Login Brothers Book Co.: *http://www.lb.com*

M
McGraw-Hill Professional Book Group: *http://books.mcgraw-hill.com/*
Merck Publications: *http://www.merck.com/!!rUN8D0IgPrUN8a0ecS/pubs/*
Mosby: *http://ww.mosby.com/*

P
Paediatric Ultrasound: *http://home.pacific.net.au/~alholley/*

S
Springer-Verlag: *http://www.springer.de/*
Springer-Verlag New York: *http://www.springer-ny.com/*

T
Thieme—Medical and Scientific Publishers: *http://www.thieme.com/*

W
W.B. Saunders: *http://www.wbsaunders.com/*

Associations/Centers

Academy of Radiology Research: www.acadrad.org
The Academy of Radiology Research Web site provides the latest information on the Academy. The Academy is intended to focus attention on radiology as a discipline committed to basic and clinical research and is dedicated to the translation of research advances into higher-quality and more cost-effective patient care.

American Board of Radiology: www.theabr.org
The American Board of Radiology Web site provides interesting information for both practitioners and residents. Statistical information as well as information on examinations and certification issues is available. Information on important dates and access to the ABR newsletter is provided.

American College of Radiology: www.acr.org
The American College of Radiology Web site provides an abundance of news, regulatory, educational and opportunities for radiologists, residents and students.

American Medical Association: www.ama-assn.org
The American Medical Association Web site provides information for all medical practitioners, training physicians, and medical students, as well as other health professionals. Information on political proceedings, educational proceedings, and industrial advances is available. There are forums on ethics and nomenclature as well as meeting information and highlights of minutes from committee groups.

A

AACOM—American Association of Colleges of Osteopathic Medicine:
  http://www.aacom.org/
AAMC—Association of American Medical Colleges: *http://www.aamc.org/*
ABMS—American Board of Medical Specialties: *http://www.abms.org/*
Academy of Radiology Research: *http://www.acadrad.org/*
ACGME—American College of Graduate Medical Education:
  http://www.acgme.org/
AHA—American Hospital Association:
  http://www.hospitalconnect.com/DesktopServlet
AMA—American Medical Association Home Page: *http://www.ama-assn.org/*
American Academy of Health Physics (AAHP): *http://hps1.org/aahp*
American Association of Academic Chief Residents in Radiology:
  http://www.a3cr2.com/
American Association of Physicists in Medicine (AAPM):
  http://www.aapm.org/
American Association for Women Radiologists: *http://www.aawr.org/*
American Board of Radiology (ABR): *http://www.theabr.org/*
American College of Medical Physics: *http://www.acmp.org/*
American College of Nuclear Physicians: *http://www.acnponline.org/*
American College of Radiology: *http://www.acr.org/*
American Healthcare Radiology Administrators (AHRA):
  http://www.ahraonline.org/default.htm
American Institute of Physics: The Physics Information NETsite:
  http://www.aip.org/
American Institute of Ultrasound in Medicine (AIUM): *http://www.aium.org/*
American Medical Informatics Association: *http://www.amia.org/*
American Nuclear Society: *http://www.ans.org/*
American Radiological Nurses Association (ARNA): *http://www.arna.net/*
American Roentgen Ray Society (ARRS): *http://www.arrs.org/*
American Society of Echocardiography: *http://asecho.org*
American Society of Head and Neck Radiology (ASHNR):
  http://www.asnr.org/ashnr/
American Society of Interventional and Therapeutic Neuroradiology:
  http://www.asitn.org/
American Society of Neuroradiology: *http://www.asnr.org/*
American Society of Nuclear Cardiology: *http://www.asnc.org/*
American Society of Pediatric Neuroradiology: *http://www.asnr.org/aspnr/*

American Society of Spine Radiology (ASSR): *http://www.asnr.org/assr/*
American Society for Therapeutic Radiology and Oncology (ASTRO):
  http://www.astro.org/
Arizona Society of Echocardiography:
  http://aztec.asu.edu/medical/azse/azse0.html
Arizona Society of Nuclear Medicine: *http://www.ahsc.arizona.edu/azssnm/*
Association of Educators in Radiological Sciences: *http://www.aers.org*
Association of Program Directors in Radiology (APDR): *http://www.apdr.org/*
Association of Vascular and Interventional Radiographers: *http://www.avir.org/*
Associazione Italiana di Neuroradiologia: *http://www.ainr.it/*
Australian Institute of Radiography: *http://www.giant.net.au/air/*
Australian Institute of Ultrasound: *http://www.aiu.edu.au/*
Australasian Society for Ultrasound in Medicine:
  http://www.asum.com/au/open/home.htm
Australian Sonographers Association: *http://www.A-S-A.com.au*

B
Brain Imaging Center, Montreal Neurological Institute, McGill University:
  http://www.bic.mni.mcgill.ca/
Brain Mapping Division, University of California, Los Angeles:
  http://www.bri.ucla.edu/
Brazilian Society of Vascular and Interventional Radiology:
  http://www.sobrice.org.br
Bristol Biomedical Image Archive: *http://www.brisbio.ac.uk/*
British Society of Paediatric Radiology: *http://www.bspr.org.uk/*
British Institute of Radiology: *http://www.bir.org.uk/*
British Medical Ultrasound Society: *http://www.bmus.org/*
British Nuclear Medicine Society: *http://www.bnms.org.uk/*

C
Canadian Association of Radiologists: *http://www.car.ca/*
Cardiovascular and Interventional Radiological Society of Europe:
  http://www.cirse.org/
Center for Biomedical Imaging Technology, University of Connecticut:
  http://www.cbit.uchc.edu/
Center for Devices and Radiological Health (CDRH):
  http://www.fda.gov/cdrh/index.html
Center for Functional Imaging, Lawrence Berkeley National Laboratory:
  http://imasun.lbl.gov/
Center for Functional Neuroimaging, University College London:
  http://www.ucl.ac.uk/CFN/
Center for Human Simulation, University of Colorado:
  http://www.uchsc.edu/sm/chs/
Center for Image Processing and Integrated Computing (CIPIC), University of
  California, Davis: *http://info.cipic.ucdavis.edu/*

Center for Imaging Science, Washington University: *http://cis.wustl.edu/*
Center for Magnetic Resonance, University of Minnesota:
  http://www.cmrr.umn.edu/
Center of Medical Imaging Research, University of Leeds:
  http://www.comp.leeds.ac.uk/comir/comir.html
Center for Molecular Imaging Research, Massachusetts General Hospital:
  http://www.mgh-cmir.org/
Center for Morphometric Analysis, Massachusetts General Hospital:
  http://dem0nmac.mgh.harvard.edu/cma/cma.homepage.html
Center for Research and Applications in Image and Signal Processing
  (CREATIS): *http://creatis-www.insa-lyon.fr/*
Center for Structural Biology, University of Florida:
  http://csbnmr.health.ufl.edu/~binglis/nmr.html
Center for X-Ray Optics: *http://www-cxro.lbl.gov/*
Centre d'Imagerie Diagnostique: *http://www.cid.ch/*
Clinical Magnetic Resonance Society: *http://www.cmrs.com/*
Clinical PET Center, Guy's and St Thomas' Hospital:
  http://www-pet.umds.ac.uk/pet-home.html
CYCERON PET Research Center: *http://www.cyceron.fr/*

D
Danish Society of Physiology and Nuclear Medicine: *http://www.dskfnm.dk/*
Danish Society of Radiology: *http://www.drs.dk*
Diagnostische Radiologie, Ernst-Moritz-Arndt-Universität Greifswald:
  http://www.uni-greifswald.de/indexuk.html
Digital Image Processing, University of Cape Town:
  http://www.dip.ee.uct.ac.za/
Digital Image Processing Laboratory, University of Michigan:
  http://www.med.umich.edu/dipl
Digital Imaging Group, Charles Sturt University:
  http://www.csu.edu.au/faculty/health/medrad/dig
Digital Imaging Unit, University Hospital of Geneva:
  http://www.expasy.ch/www.UIN/UIN.html
Division of Imaging, Westmead Hospital:
  http://www.usyd.edu.au/su/radiology/usindex.htm
Division of Physiological Imaging, Department of Radiology, University of
  Iowa College of Medicine: *http://everest.radiology.uiowa.edu/*
Dotter Interventional Institute: *http://www.ohsu.edu/dotter/dothome.html*

E
Eastern Neuroradiological Society (ENRS):
  http://www.asnr.org/etc/otherorgs/enrs1.asp
EchoWeb: Canadian Society of Echocardiography: *http://www.echoweb.org/*
Electronic Radiology Laboratory, Washington University:
  http://wuerlim.wustl.edu/

Eufora: *http://www.devolder.be/eufora*

EuroPACS: *http://www.europacs.org/ephomepage.html*

European Congress of Radiology: *http://www.ecr.org*

European Society of Head and Neck Radiology:
  http://www.eshnr.org/main.php

European Society of Neuroradiology: *http://www.esnr.org/*

European Society for Therapeutic Radiology and Oncology:
  http://www.estro.be/

European Society of Thoracic Imaging: *http://www.esti-society.org/*

F

Florida Radiological Society: *http://www.flrad.org/*

Frederik Philips Magnetic Resonance Research Center:
  http://www.emory.edu/RADIOLOGY/MRI/FPMRRCb.html

French Society of Radiology: *http://www.sfr-radiologie.asso.fr/*

H

Health Physics Society: *http://www.hps.org*

I

Imaging Research Center, Cinncinati Children's Hospital:
  http://www.irc.chmcc.org/index.html

International Society of Radiographers and Rad Technologists:
  http://www.isrrt.org/

Institut Klinische Radiologie der Westflischen Wilhelms University:
  http://medweb.uni-muenster.de/institute/ikr/

Institute of Physics: *http://www.iop.org/*

Institute of Physics and Engineering in Medicine: *http://www.ipem.org.uk/*

Institute of Radiology, University of Palermo:
  http://www.unipa.it/~radpa/radpa.html

Instituto Goiano de Radiologia: *http://www.igr.com.br*

International Radiation Protection Association (IRPA): *http://www.irpa.net/*

International Society for Magnetic Resonance in Medicine:
  http://www.ismrm.org/

International Society of Magnetic Resonance in Medicine, British Chapter:
  http://www-ipg.umds.ac.uk/ismrm-bc/

International Society of Radiographers and Rad Technologists:
  http://www.isrrt.org/

International Society of Radiology: *http://www.isradiology.org/*

Italian Society of Radiology: *http://www.sirm.org/uk/index.html*

J

Japan Radiological Society: *http://www.radiology.or.jp/*

Japan Society of Magnetic Resonance in Medicine:
   http://wwwsoc.nii.ac.jp.jmrm/
Jefferson Ultrasound Institute, Thomas Jefferson University:
   http://jeffline.tju.edu/ultrasound
Joint Center for Radiation Therapy (JCRT), Harvard Medical Center:
   http://www.jcrt.harvard.edu/jcrt/

L

Laboratory of Neuro Imaging, University of California, Los Angeles:
   http://www.loni.ucla.edu/
Levit Radiologic-Pathologic Institute:
   http://www.mdanderson.org/departments/LevitRPI/
Los Angeles Radiological Society: *http://www.larad.org*

M

Magnetic Resonance Laboratory, University of California, San Francisco:
   http://picasso.ucsf.edu//
Mallinckrodt Institute of Radiology: *http://www.mir.wustl.edu/*
MAX-Lab, Lund University, Sweden: *http://www.maxlab.lu.se/*
Medical Image Analysis: *http://www.elsevier.nl/locate/medima/*
Medical Image Format FAQ: *http://www.dclunie.com/medical-image-faq/html/*
Medical Image Perception Society:
   http://www.radiology.arizona.edu/krupinski/mips/
Medical Image Processing Group, University of Pennsylvania:
   http://www.mipg.upenn.edu/
Medical Image Processing Laboratory, State University of New York at Stony
   Brook: *http://www.mipl.rad.sunysb.edu/mipl/*
Medical Images, Shimane Medical University:
   http://www.shimane-med.ac.jp/IMAGE/IMAGE.HTM
Medical Imaging Center, Martindale's Health Science Guide:
   http://www-sci.lib.uci.edu/HSG/Medical.html
Medical Imaging Center, Turku University Central Hospital:
   http://www.utu.fi/med/radiology/mic
Medical Imaging Internet Resources:
   http://www.comp.leeds.ac.uk/comir/resources/links.html
Medical Imaging Lab, Johns Hopkins University:
   http://www.mri.jhu.edu/main.html
Medical Imaging Program, University of Virginia:
   http://imaging.med.virginia.edu/
Medical Imaging Research Group, Vancouver, B.C.:
   http://kepler.physics.ubc.ca/~mirg/
Michigan Radiological Society: *http://www.michigan-rad.org/*
Montchoisi Radiology Institute:
   http://www.montchoisi.ch/radiologie/RadiologieE.html
Musculoskeletal Ultrasound Society: *http://www.musoc.com/index.htm*

N

National Association of Portable X-Ray Providers, U.S.: *http://www.napxp.org/*
National Brain Tumor Radiosurgery Association, U.S.:
  http://www.med.jhu.edu/radiosurgery/nbtra/
National High Magnetic Field Laboratory, U.S.: *http://www.magnet.fsu.edu/*
National Institute of Radiological Sciences, Japan:
  http://www.nirs.go.jp/ENG/nirs.htm
Naval Surface Warfare Center Dahlgren Division (NSWCDD):
  http://www.nswc.navy.mil/
New Mexico Institute of Neuroimaging:
  http://www.irlen.com/research_levine.htm
New York Roentgen Society: *http://www.nyrs.org/*
New York State Radiological Society:
  http://www.informatics.sunysb.edu/nysrs/
NMR Imaging Laboratory, University of Texas, Austin:
  http://www.pe.utexas.edu/Dept/Labs/MRI/mri.html
Nordic Radiation Protection Society: *http://www.nsfs.org/nsfshomepage.html*
North American Society for Cardiac Imaging: *http://www.nasci.org*
Northeastern Ohio Association of Vascular and Interventional Radiographers:
  http://members.aol.com/znarfw/index.html
Nuclear Medicine Research Group, University of Arizona:
  http://www.ece.cmu.edu/research/radgroup/SPIE/body.html

O

Oxford Centre for Functional Magnetic Resonance Imaging of the Brain:
  http://www.fmrib.ox.ac.uk/index_r.html

P

Physics Laboratory, National Institute of Standards and Technology:
  http://physics.nist.gov/
Pitt Chemistry X-ray Crystallography Lab, University of Pittsburgh:
  http://www.pitt.edu/~geib/Welcome.html

R

Radiation Calibration Laboratory, University of Washington, Madison:
  http://uwrcl.medphysics.wisc.edu:80/
Radiation and Health Physics Home Page: *http://www.umich.edu/~radinfo/*
Radiological Research Laboratory, Stanford University:
  http://www-radiology.stanford.edu/research/
Radiological Service Training Institute: *http://www.rsti-training.com/*
Radiological Society of North America: *http://www.rsna.org/*
Radiological Society of Rhode Island (RSRI): *http://www.rirad.org/*
Radiological Society of South Africa: *http://www.rssa.co.za/*
Radiology Business Management Association (RBMA): *http://www.rbma.org/*

Radiology Imaging Research Center, University of Texas, Southwestern:
 http://www-mri.swmed.edu/
Royal Belgian Radiological Society: *http://www.rbrs.org*

S

Sociedad Nuclear España: *http://www.sne.es/*
Societé Francaise de Radiologie: *http://www.sfr-radiologie.asso.fr/*
Society for Cardiac Angiography and Interventions: *http://www.scai.org/*
Society of Cardiovascular and Interventional Radiology: *http://www.scvir.org*
Society for Cardiovascular Magnetic Resonance: *http://www.scmr.org/*
Society of Computed Body Tomography and Magnetic Resource:
 http://www.scbtmr.org
Society for Computer Applications in Radiology: *http://www.scarnet.org/*
Society of Diagnostic Medical Sonographers: *http://www.sdms.org/*
Society of Gastrointestinal Radiologists: *http://www.sgr.org/sgr.htm*
Society of Nuclear Medicine: *http://www.snm.org/*
Society of Nuclear Medicine, Southern California Chapter: *http://nucgang.org*
Society of Nuclear Medicine, Taiwan: *http://www.snm.org.tw/*
Society for Pediatric Radiology: *http://www.pedrad.org/*
Society of Radiologists in Ultrasound: *http://www.sru.org/*
Society of Radiology Oncology Administrators: *http://www.sroa.org/*
Society of Skeletal Radiology: *http://www.skeletalrad.org*
Society of Thoracic Radiology: *http://www.thoracicrad.org/*
Southeastern Neuroradiology Society (SENRS):
 http://www.asnr.org/etc/otherorgs/senrs.html
Spanish Nuclear Medicine Society: *http://www.semn.es*
Spanish Society of Vascular and Interventional Radiology:
 http://www.servei.org
Synchrotron Radiation Research Center: *http://www.srrc.gov.tw/eng/index.html*

T

Texas Radiological Society: *http://www.txrad.org/*
Turku PET Center: *http://www.utu.fi:80/med/pet/*

U

Ultrasound Research Laboratory, Mayo Clinic:
 http://www.mayo.edu/ultrasound/ultrasound.html

V

Vocal Tract Visualization Laboratory, University of Maryland:
 http://speech.umaryland.edu/

W

Western Neuroradiological Society:
 http://www.asnr.org/etc/otherorgs/wnrs.html

Wolfson Brain Imaging Center, Cambridge University:
http://www.wbic.cam.ac.uk/

Patient Resources

Radiology Resource: www.radiologyresource.org
Radiology Resource is a joint effort by the ACR and the RSNA to provide radiology-centric information to patients. The Web site provides information on all imaging studies from ultrasound to MRI. There also are sections devoted to information specially on radiologists and a glossary of terms to help patients navigate the world of medical imaging.

Med Expert: www.medexpert.net
Med Expert.net provides medical information to patients on a variety of radiology studies, from interventional to plain film chest x-rays. Many of the links provide images as well as allow patients to ask "the doctor" a question.

Virtual Hospital Information: http://www.vh.org/Patients/IHB/ DiagnosticRad.html
The Virtual Hospital Information Web site provides information for patients about popular imaging studies from an upper GI series to MRI. Information is available from why a study is performed to how it is performed to what to expect during the examination.

D
Diagnostic Radiology, Patient Information by Department, Virtual Hospital:
http://www.vh.org/Patients/IHB/DiagnosticRad.html

M
MedExpert.net: *http://www.medexpert.net/*

N
NUCMEDNET: *http://www.nucmednet.com/*

P
Patient Info. Mid-Shouth Imaging and Therapeutics:
http://www.msit.com/patients.htm
Patient Information: Diagnostic Radiology, Virtual Hospital:
http://www.vh.org/Patients/IHB/DiagnosticRad.html

R
Radiology Resource: *http://www.radiologyresource.org*

U
Ultrasound. Ask NOAH About: Pregnancy:
http://www.noah-health.org/english/pregnancy/pregnancy.html

Portals

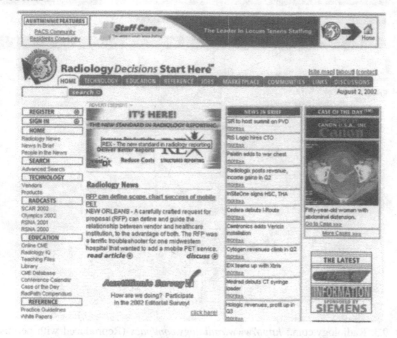

FIGURE 9.1. Auntminnie.com.: *http://www.auntminnie.com/* (Reproduced with permission from auntminnie.com.)

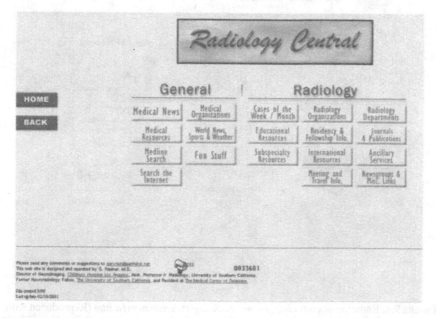

FIGURE 9.2. RadCentral.com.: *http://www.radcentral.com/* (Reproduced with permission from radcentral.com.)

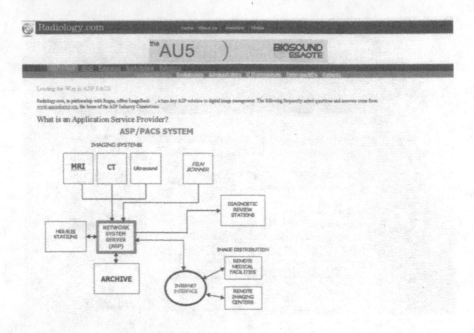

FIGURE 9.3. Radiology.com.: *http://www.radiology.com/pacs* (Reproduced with permission from radiology.com.)

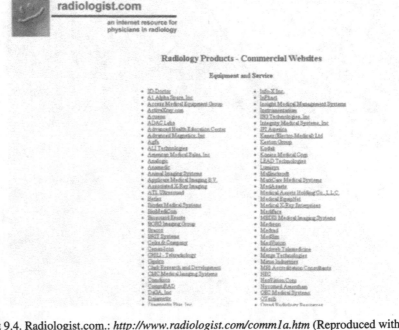

FIGURE 9.4. Radiologist.com.: *http://www.radiologist.com/comm1a.htm* (Reproduced with permission from radiologist.com.)

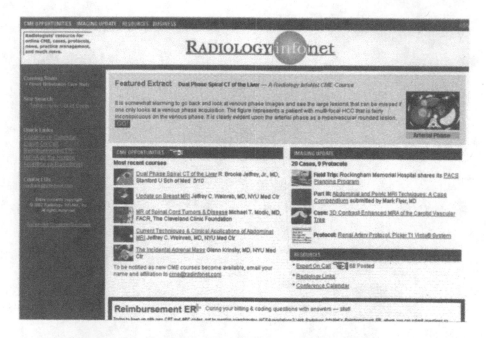

FIGURE 9.5. RadInfoNet.com.: *http://www.radinfonet.com/* (Reproduced with permission from radinfonet.com.)

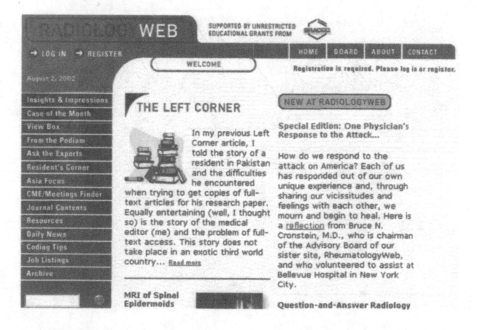

FIGURE 9.6. RadiologyWeb.: *http://www.radiologyweb.com/* (Reproduced with permission from radiologyweb.com.)

Part V
Appendices

Appendix 1

The American College of Radiology, with more than 30,000 members, is the principal organization of radiologists, radiation oncologists, and clinical medical physicists in the United States. The College is a nonprofit professional society whose primary purposes are to advance the science of radiology, improve radiologic services to the patient, study the socioeconomic aspects of the practice of radiology, and encourage continuing education for radiologists, radiation oncologists, medical physicists, and persons practicing in allied professional fields.

The American College of Radiology will periodically define new standards for radiologic practice to help advance the science of radiology and to improve the quality of service to patients throughout the United States. Existing standards will be reviewed for revision or renewal, as appropriate, on their fifth anniversary or sooner, if indicated.

Each standard, representing a policy statement by the College, has undergone a thorough consensus process in which it has been subjected to extensive review, requiring the approval of the Commission on Standards and Accreditation as well as the ACR Board of Chancellors, the ACR Council Steering Committee, and the ACR Council. The standards recognize that the safe and effective use of diagnostic and therapeutic radiology requires specific training, skills, and techniques, as described in each document.

Reproduction or modification of the published standard by those entities not providing these services is not authorized.

ACR STANDARD FOR DIGITAL IMAGE DATA MANAGEMENT

I.   INTRODUCTION AND DEFINITION

Increasingly, medical imaging and patient information are being managed utilizing digital data during acquisition, transmission, storage, display, interpretation, and consultation. The management of these data, during each of these operations, may have an impact on the quality of patient care.

These guidelines are applicable to any system of image data management, from a single modality or single-use system to a complete picture archiving and communication system. (PACS).

This standard defines goals, qualifications of personnel, equipment guidelines, specifications of data manipulation and management, and quality control and quality improvement procedures for the use of digital image data which should result in high-quality radiological care.

In all cases for which an American College of Radiology (ACR) standard exists for the modality being used or the specific examination being performed, that standard will continue to apply when digital image data management systems are used. A glossary of commonly used terminology (Appendix A) and a reference list are included.

II.   GOALS

The goals of digital image data management include, but are not limited to:

A.   Initial acquisition or generation and recording of accurately labeled and identified image data;

B.   Transmission of data to an appropriate storage medium from which it can be retrieved for display for formal interpretation, review, and consultation;

C.   Retrieval of data from available prior imaging studies to be displayed for comparison with a current study;

D.   Transmission of data to remote sites for consultation, review, or formal interpretation;

E.   Appropriate compression of image data to facilitate transmission or storage, without loss of clinically significant information;

F.   Archiving of data to maintain accurate patient medical records in a form that:

1.   May be retrieved in a timely fashion;
2.   Meets applicable facility, state, and federal regulations; and
3.   Maintains patient confidentiality.

G. Appropriate database management procedures applicable to all of the above should be in place.

It is anticipated that the goals of digital image data management will continue to evolve.

III.   QUALIFICATIONS AND RESPONSIBILITIES OF PERSONNEL

A. Physician

1. Physicians utilizing the image data management system for official interpretation[1] should understand the basic technology of image acquisition, transmission, manipulation, retrieval, and display, including the strengths, weaknesses, and limitations of these processes. Where appropriate, the interpreting physician must be familiar with the principles of radiation protection, the hazards of radiation exposure to both patients and radiological personnel, and patient and personnel monitoring requirements. The physician performing the official interpretation must be responsible for the quality of the images being reviewed and understand the elements of quality control of digital image management systems.[2]

2. The physician must demonstrate qualifications as delineated in the appropriate ACR standard for the particular diagnostic modality being interpreted.

3. The physician should have a working knowledge of those portions of the image data management system with which he/she must routinely interact, including potential technical artifacts that may result from digital image processing.

B. Technologist

1. Be certified by the appropriate registry and/or possess unrestricted state licensure;

2. Meet the qualification requirements of any existing ACR standard for acquisition of a particular examination; and

---

[1]ACR Medical Legal Committee defines official interpretation as that written report (and any supplements or amendments thereto) that attach to the patient's permanent record. In healthcare facilities with a privilege delineation system, such a written report is prepared only by a qualified physician who has been granted specific delineated clinical privileges for that purpose by the facility's governing body upon the recommendation of the medical staff.

[2]The ACR Rules of Ethics state: "It is proper for a diagnostic radiologist to provide a consultative opinion on radiographs and other images regardless of their origin. A diagnostic radiologist should regularly interpret radiographs and other images only when the radiologist reasonably participates in the quality of medical imaging, utilization review and matters of policy which affect the quality of patient care."

3.   Be trained to properly operate those portions of the image data management system with which he/she must routinely interact.

C.   Electronic/Computer Assistant

Assistants should be trained to properly operate those portions of the image data management system with which they must routinely interact.

It is desirable to have a medical physicist or image management specialists available as consultants.

D.   Medical Physicist

A Qualified Medical Physicist is an individual who is competent to practice independently one or more of the subfields in medical physics. The American College of Radiology considers that certification and continuing education in the appropriate subfield(s) demonstrate that an individual is competent to practice one or more of the subfields in medical physics and to be a Qualified Medical Physicist. The ACR recommends that the individual be certified in the appropriate subfield(s) by the American Board of Radiology (ABR).

The appropriate subfields of medical physics are: Therapeutic Radiological Physics, Diagnostic Radiological Physics, Medical Nuclear Physics, and Radiological Physics.

The continuing education of a qualified medical physicist should be in accordance with the ACR Standard for Continuing Medical Education (CME).

E.   Image Management Specialists

1.   The image management specialist should be an individual who is qualified to assess and provide problem solving input, initiate repair, and coordinate system-wide maintenance programs to assure sustainable high image quality and system function. This individual would also be directly involved with any system expansion programs.
2.   This specialist, as well as any necessary support personnel, should be available in a timely manner in case of malfunction to facilitate return to optimal system functionality.

IV.   EQUIPMENT SPECIFICATIONS

Specifications for equipment utilized in digital image data management will vary depending on the individual facility's needs but in all cases should provide image quality and availability appropriate to the clinical need whether that need be official interpretation or secondary review.

Compliance with the ACR-NEMA (National Electrical Manufacturers Association) Digital Imaging and Communications in Medicine Standard (DICOM) is strongly recommended for all new equipment acquisitions, and consideration of periodic upgrades incorporating the expanding features of that standard should be part of the ongoing quality-control program.

Equipment guidelines cover two basic categories of digital image data when used for rendering the official interpretation: small matrix size (e.g., computed tomography [CT], magnetic resonance imaging [MRI]. ultrasound, nuclear medicine and digital fluorography, digital angiography) and large matrix size (e.g., computed radiography and digitized radiographic films).

Small matrix: A data set should provide full-resolution data (typically 512 × 512 resolution at a minimum 8-bit depth) for processing, manipulation. and subsequent display.

Large matrix: A data set allowing a minimum of 2.5 lp/min spatial resolution at the original detector plane (typically 1024 × 1024 or higher resolution at a minimum 10-bit depth) for processing, manipulation, and display.

A.   Acquisition or Digitization

Initial image acquisition should be performed in accordance with the appropriate ACR modality or examination standard.

1.   Direct Image Capture
     The image data set produced on the digital modality both in terms of image matrix size and pixel bit depth should be transferred to the image management system. It is recommended that the DICOM standard be used if at all possible. This is the most desirable mode of digital image acquisition for primary diagnosis.

2.   Secondary Image Capture
     a.   Small-matrix images: Each individual image should be digitized to a matrix size as large as or larger than that of the original image on the imaging modality. The images should be digitized to a bit depth of 8 bits per pixel or greater. Film digitization or video frame grab systems conforming to the above specifications are acceptable.
     b.   Large-matrix images: These images should be digitized to a matrix size corresponding to 2.5 lp/mm or greater in the original detector plane. These images should be digitized to a bit depth of 10 bits per pixel or greater. Film digitizers will generally be required to produce these digital images.

3.   General Requirements
     At the time of acquisition (small or large matrix), the system must include:

Annotation capabilities including patient name, identification number, date and time of examination, name of facility or institution of acquisition, type of examination, patient or anatomic part orientation (i.e., right, left, superior, inferior, etc.), and amount and method of data compression.

The ability to record a brief patient history is desirable.

B. Compression

Data compression may be performed to facilitate transmission and storage. Several methods, including both reversible and irreversible techniques, may be used under the direction of a qualified physician, with no reduction in clinical diagnostic image quality. The types and ratios of compression used for different imaging studies transmitted and stored by the system should be selected and periodically reviewed by the responsible physician to ensure appropriate clinical image quality.

C. Transmission

The type and specifications of the transmission devices used will be dictated by the environment of studies to be transmitted. In all cases, for official interpretation, the digital data received at the receiving end of any transmission must have no loss of clinically significant information. The transmission system shall have adequate error-checking capability.

D. Display Capabilities

General: Display workstations used for official interpretation and for small-matrix and large-matrix systems should provide the following characteristics:

1. Luminance of the gray-scale monitors should be at least 50 foot-lamberts.
2. Care should be taken to control the lighting in the reading room to eliminate reflections in the monitor and to lower the ambient lighting level as much as is feasible.
3. Provide capability for selection of image sequence.
4. Capable of accurately associating the patient and study demographic characterizations with the study images.
5. Capable of window and level adjustment if those data are available.
6. Pan functions and zoom (magnification) functions capable of meeting guidelines for display of all acquired data.
7. Capable of rotating or flipping the images, provided labeling of patient orientation is preserved.

8. Capable of calculating and displaying accurate linear measurements and pixel value determinations in values appropriate for the modality (e.g., Hounsfield units for CT images), if those data are available.
9. Capable of displaying prior image compression ratio, processing, or cropping.
10. Elements of display that should be available include:
    a. Matrix size;
    b. Bit depth; and
    c. Total number of images acquired in the study.

E. Archiving and Retrieval

1. Digital imaging data management systems should provide storage capacity capable of complying with all facility, state, and federal regulations regarding medical record retention. Images stored at either site should meet the jurisdictional requirements of the transmitting site. Images interpreted off-site need not be stored at the receiving facility provided they are stored at the transmitting site. However, if the images are retained at the receiving site, the retention period of that jurisdiction must be met as well. The policy on record retention should be in writing.
2. Each exam data file must have an accurate corresponding patient and examination database record which includes patient name, identification number, exam date, type of examination, and facility at which the examination was performed. It is desirable that space be available for a brief clinical history.
3. Prior examinations should be retrievable from archives in a time frame appropriate to the clinical needs of the facility and medical staff.
4. Each facility should have policies and procedures for archiving and storage of digital image data equivalent to the policies that currently exist for the protection of hard-copy storage media to preserve imaging records.

F. Security

Digital image data management systems should provide network and software security protocols to protect the confidentiality of patients' identification and imaging data. There should be measures to safeguard the data and to ensure data integrity against intentional or unintentional corruption of the data.

G. Reliability and Redundancy

Quality patient care depends on availability of the digital image data management system. Written policies and procedures should be in place to ensure continuity of care at a level consistent with those for hard-copy imaging studies and medical records within a facility or institution. This should include internal redundancy systems, backup telecommunication links, and a disaster plan.

V.   DOCUMENTATION

Physicians officially interpreting examinations[3] using digital image data management systems should render reports in accordance with the ACR Standard on Communication: Diagnostic Radiology.

If reports are incorporated into the data management system. they should be retrievable with the same conditions of timeliness and security as the imaging data.

VI.   QUALITY CONTROL AND IMPROVEMENT, SAFETY, INFECTION CONTROL, AND PATIENT EDUCATION CONCERNS

Policies and procedures related to quality, patient education, infection control, and safety should be developed and implemented in accordance with the ACR Policy on Quality Control and Improvement, Safety, Infection Control, and Patient Education Concerns appearing elsewhere in this publication.

Any facility using a digital image data management system must have documented policies and procedures for monitoring and evaluating the effective management, safety, and proper performance of acquisition, digitization, compression, transmission, archiving, and retrieval functions of the system. The quality control program should be designed to maximize the quality and accessibility of diagnostic information.

A test image, such as the SMPTE test pattern[4] should be captured, transmitted, archived, retrieved, and displayed at appropriate intervals. but at least monthly, to test the overall operation of the system under conditions that simulate the normal operation of the system. As a spatial resolution test, at least 512×512 resolution should be confirmed for small-matrix official interpretation and 25 lp/mm resolution for large-matrix official interpretation.

As a test of the display, SMPTE pattern data files sized to occupy the full area used to display images on the monitor should be displayed. The overall SMPTE image appearance should be inspected to assure the absence of gross artifacts (e.g., blurring or bleeding of bright display areas into dark areas or aliasing of

---

[3]ACR Medical Legal Committee defines official interpretation as that written report (any and supplements or amendments thereto) that attach to the patient's permanent record. In health care facilities with a privilege delineation system, such a written report is prepared only by a qualified physician who has been granted specific delineated clinical privileges for that purpose by the facility's governing body upon the recommendation of the medical staff.

[4]SMPTB test pattern RP 133-1991 Gray JF, Lisk KG, Haddick DH, Harshberger JH, Oosetehof A, Schwenker R. Test pattern for video displays and hard copy cameras. Radiology 1985; 154:519-527.

spatial resolution patterns). All display monitors should be tested at least monthly. As a dynamic range test, both the 5% and the 95% areas should be seen as distinct from the respective adjacent 0% and 100% areas.

The use of digital imaging and digital image data management systems does not reduce the responsibilities for the management and supervision of radiologic examinations.

ACKNOWLEDGEMENTS

This Standard was developed according to the process described elsewhere in this publication by the Standards and Accreditation Committee of the Commission on General and Pediatric Radiology.

Principal Drafter: William T. Thorwarth, Jr., MD

William T. Thorwarth, Jr., MD, Chair
Michael C. Beachley. MD
James H. Chapman, MD
Harris L. Cohen, MD
Edmund A. Franken, MD
Howard Harcke, Jr., MD
John I. Hughes, MD
George H. Kamp, MD
William H. McAlister, MD
Thomas L. Pope, Jr., MD
William R. Reinus, MD
Stuart Royal, MS, MD
Paul Shyn, MD
Cynthia C. Youree, MD

J. Bruce Hauser, MD, CSC

REFERENCES

1. Bidgood WD Jr, Horli SC. Modular extension of the ACR-NEMA DICOM standard to support new diagnostic imaging modalities and services. J Digit Imaging 1996; 9:67-77.
2. Blaine GJ, Cox JR, Jost RG. Networks for electronic radiology. Radiol Clin North Am 1996; 34:505-524.
3. Braunschweig R, Klose HJ, Neugebauer B, et al. Digital radiography. Results of a survey (part A) and a consensus conference (part B). Bur J Radiol 1997; 7:94-101.
4. Busch HP. Digital radiography for clinical applications. Eur J Radiol 1997; 7:66-72.
5. Deibel SR, Greenes RA. Radiology systems architecture. Radiol Clin North Am 1996; 34:681-696.

6. Dwyer SJ. Imaging system architectures for picture archiving and communication systems. Radiol Clin North Am 1996; 34:495-503.
7. Horii SC. Image acquisition. Sites, technologies, and approaches. Radiol Clin North Am 1996; 34:469-494.
8. Langlotz CP, Seshadri S. Technology assessment methods for radiology systems. Radiol Clin North Am 1996; 34:667-679.
9. Lou SL, Huang HK, Arenson RL. Workstation design. Image manipulation, image set handling, and display issues. Radiol Clin North Am 1996; 34:525-544.
10. Prokop M, Schaefer-Prokop CM. Digital image processing. Eur J Radiol 1997; 7:73-82.
11. Sargent TA, Kay MG, Sargent RG. A methodology for optimally designing console panels for use by a single operator. Hum Factors 1997; 39:389-409.
12. Wang J, Langer S. A brief review of human perception factors in digital displays for picture archiving and communications systems. J Digit Imaging 1997; 10:158-168.

APPENDIX A

Glossary

Analog signal - a form of information transmission in which the signal varies in a continuous manner and is not limited to discrete steps.

Archive - a repository for digital medical images in a PACS, typically with a specific purpose of providing either short-term or long-term (permanent) storage of images. Erasable or nonerasable media may be utilized in an archive.

Baud - the number of events processed in 1 second, usually expressed in kilobits per second (kbps). Typical rates are 14.4 kbps, 28.8 kbps, and 56 kbps.

Bit (Binary digit) - the smallest piece of digital information that a computing device handles. it represents off or on (0 or 1). All data in computing devices are processed as bits or strings of bits.

Bit depth - the number of bits used to encode each pixel of the image.

Bits per second - see Throughput, Baud.

Byte - a grouping of 8 bits used to represent a character or value.

Carrier - see Data carrier.

CCD (charge-coupled device) - a photoelectric device that converts light information into electronic information. CCDs are commonly used in television cameras and image scanners and consist of an array of sensors that collect and store light as a buildup of electrical charge. The resulting electrical signal can be converted into digital values and processed digitally in a computer to form an im age.

CCD scanner - a device that uses a CCD sensor to convert film images into electronic data.

Clock - a component in a computer's processor that supplies an oscillating signal used for timing command execution and information handling.

Clock speed - the rate at which the clock oscillates or cycles. Clock speed is expressed in MHz, equal to 1 million clock cycles per second.

Compression ratio - the ratio of the number of bits in an original image to that in a compressed version of that image. For example, a compression ratio of 2:1 would correspond to a compressed image with one-half the number of bits of the original.

Consultation system - a teleradiology system used to determine the completeness of examinations, to discuss findings with other physicians, or for other applications with the knowledge that the original images will serve as the basis for the final official interpretation rendered at some later time by the physician responsible for that report.

Co-processor - a device in a computer to which specialized processing operations are delegated, such as mathematical computation or video display. The advantage of a coprocessor is that it significantly increases processing speed.

CPU (central processing unit) - the device in a computer that performs the calculations. It executes instructions (the program) and performs operations on data.

CR (computed radiography) - a system that uses a storage phosphor plate contained in a cassette instead of a film-screen cassette. A laser beam scans the exposed plate to produce the digital data that is then converted into an image.

CRT (cathode ray tube) - refers to the monitor or display device in the teleradiology system.

Data carrier - the signal that is used to transmit the data. If this signal is not present, there can be no data communication between modems.

Data communication - all forms of computer information exchange. Data communication may take place between two computers in the same building via a local area network (LAN), across the country via telephone, or around the world via satellite.

Data compression - methods to reduce the data volume by encoding it in a more efficient manner, thus reducing the image processing and transmission times and storage space required. These methods may be reversible or irreversible.

Data transfer rate - the speed at which information is transferred between devices, such as a scanner and a computer; between components within a device, such as between storage and memory in a computer; or between teleradiology stations.

Dedicated line - a telephone line that is reserved for the exclusive use of one customer. It can be used 24 hours a day and usually offers better quality than a standard dial-up telephone line but may not significantly increase the performance of data communication.

DICOM (Digital Imaging and Communications in Medicine) - a standard for interconnection of medical digital imaging devices, developed and sponsored by the American College of Radiology and the National Electrical Manufacturers Association.

Digital signal - a form of information transmission in which the signal varies in discrete steps, not in a continuous manner.

Digitize - the process by which analog (continuous value) information is converted into digital (discrete value) information. This process is a necessary function for computer imaging applications because visual information is inherently in analog format and most computers use only digital information.

Direct image capture - the capture or acquisition of digital image data that has been acquired in digital format by an imaging modality. The image produced from the data, regardless of the modality that produced it, (CT, MRI, CR, US) is identical to the original.

dpi (dots per inch) - while in conventional radiography resolution is commonly expressed in line pairs per millimeter (lp/mm), film digitizer resolution is commonly expressed as dots (pixels) per inch.

Dynamic range - the ability of a communication or imaging system to transmit or reproduce a range of information or brightness values.

File - a set of digital data that have a common purpose, such as an image, a program, or a database.

Floppy diskette - a data storage device made of metal-coated plastic that can store computer information and can be physically transported from one place to another. The storage capacity of floppy diskettes is usually in the range of 360K to 1.5 MB, which is too small to be of use in imaging applications.

Floppy diskette drive - the device on a computer that can read and write to floppy diskettes. It is used to import and export data.

G (giga) - stands for the number 1 billion. It is used primarily when referring to computer storage capacities; for example, 1 GB = 1 billion bytes or 1000 megabytes.

Gray scale - the number of different shades of levels of gray that can be stored and displayed by a computer system. The number of gray levels is directly related to the number of bits used in each pixel: 6 bits = 64 gray levels, 7 bits = 128 gray levels, 8 bits = 256 gray levels, 10 bits = 1024 gray levels, and 12 bits = 4096 gray levels.

Gray-scale monitor - a black-to-white display with varying shades of gray, ranging from several shades to thousands, thus being suitable for use in imaging. This type of monitor also may be referred to as a monochrome display. (See also monochrome monitor)

Hard disk drive - an internal computer device that is used for storage of data.

Hardware - a collective term used to describe the physical components that form a computer. The monitor, CPU, disk drives, memory, modem, and other components are all considered hardware. It you can touch it, it is hardware.

HIS (hospital information system) - an integrated computer-based system to store and retrieve patient information, including laboratory and radiology reports.

IDE (integrated device electronics) - a type of interface used for hard disk drives that integrates the control electronics for the interface on the drive itself. Its purpose is to increase the speed at which information can be transferred between the hard disk and the rest of the computer.

IMACS - Image Management and Communication System.

Image - a computer's digital representation of a physical object.

Image compression - reduction of the amount of data required to represent an image. This is accomplished by encoding the spatial and contrast information more efficiently or discarding some non-essential information or both.

Interface - the connection between two computers or parts of computers. It consists mainly of electronic circuitry.

Irreversible compression - some permanent alteration of digital image data. This is sometimes referred to as lossy.

ISDN (integrated services digital network) - a switched network with end-to-end digital connection enabling copper wiring to perform functions such as high-speed transmission, which frequently requires higher capacity fiberoptic cable.

K (kilo) - stands for the number 1000. It is used primarily when referring to computer storage and memory capacities: for example, 1 kbps = 1024 bytes.

LAN (local area network) - computers in a limited area linked by cables that allow the exchange of data.

Laser film scanner - a device that uses a laser beam to convert an image on X-ray into digital image data.

Leased line - same as a dedicated line.

Lossless - see reversible compression.

Lossy - see irreversible compression.

M (mega) - stands for the number 1 million. It is used primarily when referring to computer storage and memory capacities: for example, 1 MB = 1 million bytes. 1 MB = 1024 thousand bytes or 1000 kbytes.

Matrix size:
Small - defined as images from CT, MR, ultrasound, nuclear medicine, and digital fluorography.
Large - defined as images from computed radiography, and digitized radiographic films.

Memory - electronic circuitry within a computer that stores information.

Modem - a device that converts digital signals from a computer to pulse tone signals for transmission over telephone lines.

Monochrome monitor - a computer display in which an image is presented as different shades of gray from black to white. (see also gray-scale monitor)

Mouse - an input device that allows the computer user to point to objects on the screen and execute commands.

Operating system - software that allocates and manages the resources available within a computer system. UNIX, MS-DOS, Macintosh, and Windows are examples of operating systems.

Optical disk - a computer data storage disk used primarily for large amounts (GB) of data.

PACS - Picture Archiving and Communication System.

Peripheral - a device that is connected to a computer and performs a function. Scanners, mouse pointers, printers, keyboards, and monitors are examples of peripherals.

Phosphor - the coating on the inside of a CRT or monitor that produces light when it is struck by an electron beam.

Pixel (picture element) - the smallest piece of information that can be displayed on a CRT. It is represented by a numerical code within the computer and displayed on the monitor as a dot of a specific color or intensity. An image is composed of a large array of pixels of differing intensities or colors.

Protocol - a set of guidelines by which two different computer devices communicate with each other.

RAM (random access memory) - a type of temporary memory in a computer in which programs are run, images are processed, and information is stored. The amount of RAM that a computer requires varies widely depending on the specific application. Information stored in RAM is lost when the power is shut off.

Resolution - the ability of an imaging system to differentiate between objects.

Reversible compression - no alteration of original image information upon reconstruction. This is sometimes referred to as lossless.

RIS (radiology information system)

Roam and zoom - the ability to select and magnify a region in the display.

ROM (read only memory) - a permanent memory which is an integral part of the computer. Programs and information stored in ROM are not lost when the power is removed.

SCSI (small computer systems interface) - SCSI is an interface protocol that is used to link dissimilar computer devices so that they can exchange data. SCSI interfaces are most common in image scanners and mass storage devices. This type of interface is well suited for imaging applications.

Secondary image capture - the capture in digital format of image data that originally existed in another primary format (e.g., a digital image data file on a CT scanner, or a screen-film radiographic film) through the process of video capture or film digitization.

Software - a name given to the programs or sets of programs that are executed on a computer.

Tera (T) - stands for approximately 1 trillion (10^{12}). It is used primarily when referring to archive storage capabilities; for example, 1 TB = 1 trillion bytes, 1 million MB, or 1000 GB.

Throughput - a measure of the amount of data that is actually being communicated, expressed in bits per second. It is related to the baud rate, but is usually somewhat less in value due to non-ideal circumstances. Typically, modems with higher baud rates can attain a higher throughput.

Video capture - the process by which images are digitized directly from the video display console of a modality, such as CT, MRI, or ultrasound. The video signal is converted to a digital signal. This process is more efficient and produces better quality images than scanning films that are produced by the same equipment.

Voxel (volume element, derived from pixel) - a voxel is, as the name would imply, a three-dimensional version of a pixel. Voxels are generated by computer-based imaging systems, such as CT and MRI. Using voxels, three-dimensional simulations of objects can be reconstructed by imaging systems.

WAN (wide area network) - a communication system that extends over large distances (covering more than a metropolitan area), often employing multiple communication link technologies such as copper wire, coaxial cable, and fiberoptic links. The cost of these WANS is presently dominated by transmission costs.

WORM (write once read many times) - a peripheral memory device that stores information permanently.

Appendix 2

The American College of Radiology, with more than 30,000 members, is the principal organization of radiologists, radiation oncologists, and clinical medical physicists in the United States. The College is a nonprofit professional society whose primary purposes are to advance the science of radiology, improve radiologic services to the patient, study the socioeconomic aspects of the practice of radiology. and encourage continuing education for radiologists, radiation oncologists, medical physicists, and persons practicing in allied professional fields.

The American College of Radiology will periodically define new standards for radiologic practice to help advance the science of radiology and to improve the quality of service to patients throughout the United States. Existing standards will be reviewed for revision or renewal, as appropriate, on their fifth anniversary or sooner, if indicated.

Each standard, representing a policy statement by the College, has undergone a thorough consensus process in which it has been subjected to extensive review, requiring the approval of the Commission on Standards and Accreditation as well as the ACR Board of Chancellors, the ACR Council Steering Committee, and the ACR Council. The standards recognize that the safe and effective use of diagnostic and therapeutic radiology requires specific training, skills, and techniques, as described in each document.

Reproduction or modification of the published standard by those entities not providing these services is not authorized.

ACR STANDARD FOR TELERADIOLOGY

I.   INTRODUCTION AND DEFINITION

Teleradiology is the electronic transmission of radiological images from one location to another for the purposes of interpretation and/or consultation. Teleradiology may allow more timely interpretation of radiological images and give greater access to secondary consultations and to improved continuing education. Users in different locations may simultaneously view images. Appropriately utilized, teleradiology may improve access to radiological interpretations and thus significantly improve patient care.

Teleradiology is not appropriate if the available teleradiology system does not provide images of sufficient quality to perform the indicated task. When a teleradiology system is used to produce the official interpretation, there should not be a clinically significant loss of spatial or contrast resolution from image acquisition through transmission to final image display. For transmission of images for display use only, the image quality should be sufficient to satisfy the needs of the clinical circumstance.

This standard defines goals, qualifications of personnel, equipment guidelines, licensing, credentialing, liability, communication, quality control, and quality improvement for teleradiology. While not all-inclusive, the standard should serve as a model for all physicians and health care workers who utilize teleradiology. A glossary of commonly used terminology (Appendix A) and a reference list are included.

II.   GOALS

Teleradiology is an evolving technology. New goals will continue to emerge.

The current goals of teleradiology include:

A. Providing consultative and interpretative radiological services in areas of demonstrated need;

B. Making radiologic consultations available in medical facilities without on-site radiologic support;

C. Providing timely availability of radiological images and radiological image interpretation in emergent and non-emergent clinical care areas;

D. Facilitating radiological interpretations in on-call situations;

E. Providing subspecialty radiological support as needed;

F. Enhancing educational opportunities for practicing radiologists;

G. Promoting efficiency and quality improvement;

H. Sending interpreted images to referring providers;

I. Supporting telemedicine; and

J. Providing direct supervision of off-site imaging studies.

III.   QUALIFICATIONS OF PERSONNEL

The radiological examination at the transmitting site must be performed by qualified personnel trained in the examination to be performed. In all cases this means a licensed and/or registered radiologic technologist, nuclear medicine technologist, or sonography technologist/sonographer. This technologist must be under the supervision of a qualified licensed physician.

It is desirable to have physicist and/or image management specialist on site or as consultants.

A. Physician

The official interpretation[1] of images must be done by a physician who has:

1. An understanding of the basic technology of teleradiology, its strengths and weaknesses (as well as limitations), and who is trained in the use of the teleradiology equipment.
2. Demonstrated qualifications as delineated in the appropriate American College of Radiology (ACR) standard for the particular diagnostic modality being transmitted through teleradiology.

B. Technologist

The technologist or sonographer should be:
1. Certified by the appropriate registry and/or possess unrestricted state licensure.
2. Trained to properly operate and supervise the teleradiology system.

C. Physicist

A Qualified Medical Physicist is an individual who is competent to practice independently one or more of the subfields in medical physics. The American College of Radiology considers that certification and continuing education in the appropriate subfield(s) demonstrate that an individual is competent to practice one

---

[1]ACR Medical Legal Committee defines official interpretation as that written report (and any supplements or amendments thereto) that attach to the patient's permanent record. In health are facilities with a privilege delineation system, such a written report is prepared only by a qualified physician who has been granted specific delineated clinical privileges for that purpose by the facility's governing body upon the recommendation of the medical staff.

or more of the subfields in medical physics and to be a Qualified Medical Physicist. The ACR recommends that the individual be certified in the appropriate subfield(s) by the American Board of Radiology (ABR).

The appropriate subfields of medical physics are: Therapeutic Radiological Physics, Diagnostic Radiological Physics, Medical Nuclear Physics, and Radiological Physics.

The continuing education of a qualified medical physicist should be in accordance with the ACR Standard for Continuing Medical Education (CME).

D. Image Management Specialist

1. The image management specialist should be an individual who is qualified by virtue of education and experience to assess and provide problem-solving input, initiate repair, and coordinate system-wide maintenance programs to assure sustainable high-image quality and system function. This individual would also be directly involved with any system variances and expansion programs.
2. This specialist should be available in a timely manner in case of malfunction to facilitate return to optimal system functionality.

IV.   EQUIPMENT SPECIFICATIONS

Specifications for equipment utilized in teleradiology will vary depending on the individual facility's needs but, in all cases, should provide image quality and availability appropriate to the clinical need.

Compliance with the ACR/NEMA (National Electrical Manufacturers Association) Digital Imaging and Communication in Medicine Standard (DICOM) is strongly recommended for all new equipment acquisitions and consideration of periodic upgrades incorporating the expanding features of that standard should be part of the ongoing quality-control program.

Equipment guidelines cover two basic categories of teleradiology when used for rendering the official interpretation: small matrix size (e.g., computed tomography (CT), magnetic resonance imaging (MR), ultrasound, nuclear medicine, digital fluorography, and digital angiography) and large matrix size (e.g., computed radiography and digitized radiographic films).

Small matrix: A data set should provide full-resolution data (typically 512×512 resolution at minimum 8-bit depth) for processing, manipulation, and subsequent display.

Large matrix: A data set allowing a minimum of 2.5 lp/mm spatial resolution at minimum 10-bit depth should be acquired.

A. Acquisition or Digitization

Initial image acquisition should be performed in accordance with the appropriate ACR modality or examination standard.

1. Direct image capture
    The image data set produced by the digital modality both in terms of image matrix size and pixel bit depth should be transferred to the teleradiology system. It is recommended that the DICOM standard be used. This is the most desirable mode of digital image acquisition for primary diagnosis.
2. Secondary image capture
    a. Small matrix images. Each individual image should be digitized to a matrix size as large or larger than that of the original image by the imaging modality The images should be digitized to a bit depth of 8 bits per pixel or greater. Film digitization or video frame grab systems conforming to the above specifications are acceptable.
    b. Large matrix images. These images should be digitized to a matrix size corresponding to 2.5 lp/mm or greater, measured in the original detector plane. These images should be digitized to a bit depth of 10 bits per pixel or greater. Film digitizers will generally be required to produce these digital images.
3. General requirements
    At the time of acquisition (small or large matrix), the system must include: Annotation capabilities including patient name, identification number, date and time of examination, name of facility or institution of acquisition, type of examination, patient or anatomic part orientation (e.g., right, left, superior, inferior, etc.), amount and method of data compression. The capability to record a brief patient history is desirable.

B. Compression

Data compression may be performed to facilitate transmission and storage. Several methods, including both reversible and irreversible techniques, may be used, under the direction of a qualified physician, with no reduction in clinically diagnostic image quality The types and ratios of compression used for different imaging studies transmitted and stored by the system should be selected and periodically reviewed by the responsible physician to ensure appropriate clinical image quality.

C. Transmission

The type and specifications of the transmission devices used will be dictated by the environment of the studies to be transmitted. In all cases, for official interpretation, the digital data received at the receiving end of any transmission must have no loss of clinically significant information. The transmission system shall have adequate error-checking capability.

D.   Display Capabilities

General: Display workstations used for official interpretation and employed for small matrix and large matrix systems should provide the following characteristics:

1.   Luminance of the gray-scale monitors should be at least 50 foot-lamberts;
2.   Care should be taken to control the lighting in the reading room to eliminate reflections in the monitor and to lower the ambient lighting level as much as is feasible.
3.   Provide capability for selection of image sequence;
4.   Capable of accurately associating the patient and study demographic characterizations with the study images;
5.   Capable of window and level adjustment, if those data are available;
6.   Capable of pan functions and zoom (magnification) function;
7.   Capable of meeting guidelines for display of all acquired data;
8.   Capable of rotating or flipping the images, provided correct labeling of patient orientation is preserved;
9.   Capable of calculating and displaying accurate linear measurements and pixel value determinations in appropriate values for the modality (e.g., Hounsfield units for CT images), if those data are available;
10.   Capable of displaying prior image compression ratio, processing, or cropping; and
11.   Elements of display that should be available include:
     a.   Matrix size;
     b.   Bit depth; and
     c.   Total number of images acquired in the study.

There may be less stringent guidelines for display systems when these display systems are not used for the official interpretation.

E.   Archiving and Retrieval

If electronic archiving is to be employed the guidelines listed below should be followed:

1.   Teleradiology systems should provide storage capacity capable of complying with all facility, state, and federal regulations regarding medical record retention. Images stored at either site should meet the jurisdictional requirements of the transmitting site. Images interpreted off-site need not be stored at the receiving facility, provided they are stored at the transmitting site. However, if the images are retained at the receiving site, the retention period of that jurisdiction must be met as well. The policy on record retention should be in writing.
2.   Each exam data file must have an accurate corresponding patient and examination database record, which includes patient name, identification number, exam date, type of examination, facility at which exami-

nation was performed. It is desirable that space be available for a brief clinical history.

3. Prior examinations should be retrievable from archives in a time frame appropriate to the clinical needs of the facility and medical staff.

4. Each facility should have policies and procedures for archiving and storage of digital image data equivalent to the policies that currently exist for the protection of hard-copy storage media to preserve imaging records.

F. Security

Teleradiology systems should provide network and software security protocols to protect the confidentiality of patients' identification and imaging data. There should be measures to safeguard the data and to ensure data integrity against intentional or unintentional corruption of the data.

G. Reliability and Redundancy

Quality patient care depends on availability of the teleradiology system. Written policies and procedures should be in place to ensure continuity of care at a level consistent with those for hard-copy imaging studies and medical records within a facility or institution. This should include internal redundancy systems, backup telecommunication links, and a disaster plan.

V.   LICENSING, CREDENTIALING, AND LIABILITY

Physicians who provide the official interpretation[2] of images transmitted by teleradiology should maintain licensure appropriate to delivery of radiologic service at both the transmitting and receiving sites. When providing the official interpretation of images from a hospital, the physician should be credentialed and obtain appropriate privileges at that institution. These physicians should consult with their professional liability carrier to ensure coverage in both the sending and receiving sites (state or jurisdiction).

The physician performing the official interpretations must be responsible for the quality of the images being reviewed.[3]

---

[2]ACR Medical Legal Committee defines official interpretation as that written report (and any supplements or amendments thereto) that attach to the patient's permanent record. In healthcare facilities with a privilege delineation system, such a written report is prepared only by a qualified physician who has been granted specific delineated clinical privileges for that purpose by the facility's governing body upon the recommendation of the medical staff.

[3]The ACR Rules of Ethics state: "it is proper for a diagnostic radiologist to provide a consultative opinion on radiographs and other images regardless of their origin. A diagnostic radiologist should regularly interpret radiographs and other images only when the radiologist reasonably participates in the quality of medical imaging, utilization review, and matters of policy which affect the quality of patient care."

Images stored at either site should meet the jurisdictional requirements of the transmitting site. Images interpreted off-site need not be stored at the receiving facility, provided they are stored at the transmitting site. However, if images are retained at the receiving site, the retention period of that jurisdiction must be met as well. The policy on record retention should be in writing.

The physicians who are involved in practicing teleradiology will conduct their practice in a manner consistent with the bylaws, rules, and regulations for patient care at the transmitting site.

VI.   DOCUMENTATION

Communication is a critical component of teleradiology. Physicians interpreting teleradiology examinations should render reports in accordance with the ACR Standard for Communication: Diagnostic Radiology.

VII.   QUALITY CONTROL AND IMPROVEMENT, SAFETY, INFECTION CONTROL, AND PATIENT EDUCATION CONCERNS

Policies and procedures related to quality, patient education, infection control and safety should be developed and implemented in accordance with the ACR Policy on Quality Control and Improvement, Safety, Infection Control, and Patient Education Concerns appearing elsewhere in this publication.

Any facility using a teleradiology system must have documented policies and procedures for monitoring and evaluating the effective management, safety, and proper performance of acquisition, digitization, compression, transmission, archiving, and retrieval functions of the system. The quality-control program should be designed to maximize the quality and accessibility of diagnostic information.

A test image, such as the SMPTE test pattern[4] should be captured, transmitted, archived, retrieved, and displayed at appropriate intervals, but at least monthly, to test the overall operation of the system under conditions that simulate the normal operation of the system. As a spatial resolution test, at least 512×512 resolution should be confirmed for small-matrix official interpretation, and 2.5 lp/mm resolution for large-matrix official interpretation.

---

[4]SMPTE test pattern RP 133-1991. Gray Jf, Lisk KG, Haddick DH, Harshberger JR, Oosetehof A, Sehwenker R. Test pattern for video displays and hard copy cameras. Radiology 1985; 154:519–527.

As a test of the display, SMPTE pattern data files sized to occupy the full area used to display images on the monitor should be displayed. The overall SMPTE image appearance should be inspected to assure the absence of gross artifacts (e.g., blurring or bleeding of bright display areas into dark areas or aliasing of spatial resolution patterns). Display monitors used for primary interpretation should be tested at least monthly. As a dynamic range test, both the 5% and the 95% areas should be seen as distinct from the respective adjacent 0% and 100% areas.

The use of teleradiology does not reduce the responsibilities for the management and supervision of radiologic medicine.

ACKNOWLEDGEMENTS

This Standard was revised according to the process described elsewhere in this publication by the Standards and Accreditation Committee of the Commission on General and Pediatric Radiology.

William T. Thorwarth, Jr., MD, Chair
Michael C. Beachley, MD
James H. Chapman, MD
Harris L. Cohen, MD
Edmund A. Franken, MD
Howard Harcke, Jr. MD
John J. Hughes, MD
George H. Kamp, MD
William H. McAlister, MD
Thomas L. Pope, Jr., MD
William R. Reinus, MD
Stuart Royal, MS, MD
Paul Shyn, MD
Cynthia C. Youree, MD

　　J. Bruce Hauser, MD, CSC

REFERENCES

1. Ackerman LV, Gitlin JN. ACR-NEMA Digital imaging communication standard: demonstration at RSNA '92 InfoRAD. Radiology 1992; 185:394.
2. Ackerman SJ, Gitlin JN, Gayler RW, et al. Receiver operating characteristic analysis of fracture and pneumonia detection: comparison of laser-digitized workstation images and conventional analog radiographs. Radiology 1993; 186:263-268.
3. Averch TD, O'Sullivan D, Breitenbach C, et al. Digital radiographic imaging transfer comparison with plain radiographs. J Endouro 1997; 11:99-101.

4. Barnes GT, Morin RL, Staab EV. InfoRAD: computers for clinical practice and education in radiology. Teleradiology: fundamental considerations and clinical applications. RadioGraphics 1993; 13:673-681.
5. Batnitaky S, Rosenthal SJ, Siegel EL, et al. Teleradiology: an assessment. Radiology 1990; 177:11-17.
6. Baur HJ, Engelmann U, Saurbier F, et al. How to deal with security issues in teleradiology. Comput Methods Programs Biomed 1997; 53:1-8.
7. Berger SB, Cepelewicz BB. Medical-legal issues in teleradiology. AJR 1996; 166:505-510.
8. Bidgood WD, Horii SC. Introduction to the ACR-NEMA DICOM standard. RadioGraphics 1992; 12:345-355.
9. Bidgood WD, Horii SC. Modular extension of the ACR-NEMA DICOM standard to support new diagnostic imaging modalities and services. J Digit Imaging 1996; 9:67-77.
10. Blaine GJ, Cox JR, Jost RG. Networks for electronic radiology. Radiol Clin North AM 1996; 34:505-524.
11. Bolle SR, Sund T, Stormer I. Receiver operating characteristic study of image preprocessing for teleradiology and digital workstations. J Digit Imaging 1997; 10:152-157.
12. Braunschweig R, Klose HJ, Neugebauer E, et al. Digital radiography. Results of a survey (part A) and a consensus conference (part B). Eur Radiol 1997; 3:S94-S101.
13. Brenner RJ, Westenberg L. Film management and custody: current and future medicolegal issues. AJR 1996: 67:1371-1375.
14. Brody WR, Johnston GS. Computer applications to assist radiology, SCAR '92. Symposium for Computer Assisted Radiology.
15. Busch HP. Digital radiography for clinical applications. Eur J Radiol 1997; 7:66-72.
16. Cawthon MA, Goeringer F, Telepak RJ, et al. Preliminary assessment of computed tomography and satellite teleradiology from Operation Desert Storm. Invest Radiol 1991; 26:854-857.
17. Deibel SR, Greenes RA. Radiology systems architecture. Radiol Clin North AM 1996; 34:681-696.
18. De Simone DN, Kundel HL, Arenson RL, et al. Effect of a digital imaging network on physician behavior in an intensive care unit. Radiology 1988; 169:41-44.
19. Dwyer SI III. Imaging system architectures for picture rehiving and communication systems. Radiol Clin North AM 1996; 34:495-503.
20. Dwyer SJ III, Templeton AW, Batnitzky S. Teleradiology: costs of hardware and communications. AJR 1991; 156:1279-1282.
21. Franken EA Jr, Berbaum KS. Subspecialty radiology consultation by interactive telemedicine. J Telemed Telecare 1996; 2:35-41.
22. Franken EA Jr, Berbaum KS, Smith WL, et al. Teleradiology for rural hospitals: analysis of a field study. J Telemed Telecare 1995; 1:202-208.
23. Franken EA Jr, Harkens KL, Berbaum KS. Teleradiology consultation for a rural hospital: patterns of use. Acad Radiol 1997; 4:492-496.
24. Gitlin JN. Teleradiology. Radiol Clin North Am 1986: 24:55-68.
25. Goldberg MA, Rosenthal DI, Chew FS, et al. New high-resolution teleradiology system: prospective study of diagnostic accuracy in 685 transmitted clinical cases. Radiology 1993; 186:429–434.
26. Goldberg MA. Teleradiology and telemedicine. Radiol Clin North Am 1996; 34:647-665.
27. Gray JE. Use of the SMPTE test pattern in picture archiving and communication systems. J Digit Imaging. 1992; 5:54-58.

28. Hassol A, Gaumer G, Irvin C, et al. Rural telemedicine data/image transfer methods and purposes of interactive video sessions. J Am Med Inform Assoc 1997; 4:36-37.
29. Horii SC. Image acquisition. Sites, technologies, and approaches. Radiol Clin North Am 1996; 34:469-494.
30. Kamp GH. Medical-legal issues in teleradiology: a commentary. AJR 1996; 166:511-512.
31. Kehler M, Bengtsson PO, Freitag M, et al. Teleradiology by two different concepts. Technical note. Acta Radiol 1997; 38:338-339.
32. Kelsey CA. A guide to teleradiology systems. Reston, Va: American College of Radiology, 1993.
33. Langlotz CP, Seshadri S. Technology assessment methods for radiology systems. Radiol Clin North Am 1996; 34:667-679.
34. Lou SL, Huang HK, Arenson RL. Workstation design. Image manipulation, image set handling, and display issues. Radiol Clin North Am 1996; 34:525-544.
35. Maldjian JA, Liu WC, Hirschorn D, et al. Wavelet transform-based image compression for transmission of MR data. AJR 1997; 169:23-26.
36. Mattel I, Jimenez MD, Martin-Santos FJ, et al. Accuracy of teleradiology in skeletal disorders: solitary bone lesions and fractures. J Telemed Telecare 1995; 1:13-18.
37. Prokop M, Schaefer-Prokop CM. Digital image processing. Eur J Radiol 1997; 7:73-82.
38. Sargent TA, Kay MG, Sargent RG. A methodology for optimally designing console panels for use by a single operator. Hum Factors 1997; 39:389-409.
39. Stewart. Clinical utilization of grayscale workstations. IEEE, Eng Med Biol 1993:86-102.
40. Stormer I, Bolle SR, Sund T, et al. ROC-study of a teleradiology workstation versus film readings. Acta Radiol 1997; 38:176-180.
41. Templeton AW, Dwyer SJ, Rosenthal SI, et al. A dial up digital teleradiology system: technical considerations and clinical experience. AJR 1991; 157:1331-1336.
42. Wang J, Langer S. A brief review of human perception factors in digital displays for picture archiving and communications systems. J Digit Imaging 1997; 10:158-168.
43. Whelan LI. Teleradiology legal issues. J Digit Imaging 1997; 10(Suppl 1):17-18.
44. Yamamoto LG, Ash KM, Boychuk RB, et al. Personal computer teleradiology interhospital image transmission of neonatal radiographs to facilitate tertiary neonatology telephone consultation and patient transfer. J Perinatol 1996; 16:292-298.
45. Yoo SK, Kim SR, Kim NH, et al. Design of an emergency teleradiology system based on progressive transmission. Yonsei Med J 11995; 36:426-437.

APPENDIX A

Glossary *

Analog signal - a form of information transmission in which the signal varies in a continuous manner and is not limited to discrete steps.

Archive - a repository for digital medical images in a picture archiving and communications system (PACS), typically with a specific purpose of providing either short-term or long-term (permanent) storage of images. Erasable or non-erasable media may be utilized in an archive.

Baud - the number of events processed in 1 second, usually expressed in bits per second (bps) or kilobits per second (kbps). Typical rates are 14.4 kbps, 28.8 kbps, and 56 kbps.

Bit (binary digit) - the smallest piece of digital information that a computing device handles. It represents off or on (0 or 1). All data in computing devices are processed as bits or strings of bits.

Bit depth - the number of bits used to encode each pixel of the image.

Bits per second - see Throughput, Baud.

Byte - a grouping of 8 bits used to represent a character or value.

Carrier - see Data Carrier

CCD (charge-coupled device) - a photoelectric device that converts light information into electronic information. CCDs are commonly used in television cameras and image scanners and consist of an array of sensors that collect and store light as a buildup of electrical charge. The resulting electrical signal can be converted into digital values and processed digitally in a computer to form an image.

CCD scanner - a device that uses a CCD sensor to convert film images into electronic data.

Clock - a component in a computer's processor that supplies an oscillating signal used for timing command execution and information handling.

Clock speed - the rate at which the clock oscillates or cycles. Clock speed is expressed in MHz, equal to 1 million clock ticks per second.

Compression ratio - the ratio of the number of bits in an original image to that in a compressed version of that image. For example, a compression ratio of 2:1 would correspond to a compressed image with one-half the number of bits of the original.

Consultation system - a teleradiology system used to determine the completeness of examinations, to discuss findings with other physicians, or for other applications, with the knowledge that the original images will serve as the basis for the final official interpretation rendered at some later time by the physician responsible for that report.

Co-processor - a device in a computer to which specialized processing operations are delegated such as mathematical computation or video display. The advantage of a co-processor is that it significantly increases processing speed.

CPU (central processing unit) - the device in a computer that performs the calculations. It executes instructions (the program) and performs operations on data.

CR (computed radiography) - a system that uses a storage phosphor plate contained in a cassette instead of a film-screen cassette. A laser beam scans the exposed plate to produce the digital data that is then converted into an image.

CRT (cathode ray tube) - refers to the monitor or display device in the teleradiology system.

Data carrier - the signal that is used to transmit the data. If this signal is not present, there can be no data communication between modems.

Data communication - all forms of computer information exchange. Data communication may take place between two computers in the same building via a local area network (LAN), across the country via telephone, or around the world via satellite.

Data compression - methods to reduce the data volume by encoding it in a more efficient manner, thus reducing the image processing and transmission times and storage space required. These methods may be reversible or irreversible.

Data transfer rate - the speed at which information is transferred between devices, such as a scanner and a computer; between components within a device, such as between storage and memory in a computer; or between teleradiology stations.

Dedicated lines - a telephone line that is reserved for the exclusive use of one customer. It can be used 24 hours a day and usually offers better quality than a standard dial-up telephone line but may not significantly increase the performance of data communication.

DICOM (digital imaging and communications in medicine) - a standard for interconnection of medical digital imaging devices, developed by the ACR-NEMA committee sponsored by the American College of Radiology and the National Electrical Manufacturers Association.

Digital signal - a form of information transmission in which the signal varies in discrete steps, not in a continuous manner.

Digitize - the process by which analog (continuous value) information is converted into digital (discrete value) information. This process is a necessary function for computer imaging applications because visual information is inherently in analog format and most computers use only digital information.

Direct image capture - the capture or acquisition of digital image data that have been acquired in digital format by an imaging modality. The image produced from the data, regardless of the modality that produced it (CT, MRI, computed radiography, ultrasound) is identical to the original.

dpi (dots per inch) - while in conventional radiography, resolution is commonly expressed in pairs per millimeter (lp/mm), film digitizer resolution is commonly expressed as dots (pixels) per inch.

Dynamic range - the ability of a communication or imaging system to transmit or reproduce a spectrum of information or brightness values.

File - a set of digital data that have a common purpose, such as an image, a program, or a database.

Floppy diskette - a data storage device made of metal-coated plastic that can store computer information and can be physically transported from one place to another. The storage capacity of floppy diskettes is usually in the range of 360 K to 1.5 megabytes, which is too small to be of use in imaging applications.

Floppy diskette drive - the device on a computer that can read and write to floppy diskettes. It is used to import and export data.

G (giga) - stands for the number 1 billion. It is used primarily when referring to computer storage capacities; for example, 1 GB = 1 billion bytes or 1000 megabytes.

Gray scale - the number of different shades of levels of gray that can be stored and displayed by a computer system. The number of gray levels is directly related to the number of its used in each pixel: 6 bits = 64 gray levels, 7 bits = 128 gray levels, 8 bits = 256 gray levels, 10 bits = 1024 gray levels, and 12 bits = 4096 gray levels.

Gray-scale monitor - a black-to-white display with varying shades of gray, ranging from several shades to thousands, thus being suitable for use in imaging. This type of monitor also may be referred to as a monochrome display. (see also monochrome monitors)

Hard disk drive - an internal computer device that is used for storage of data.

Hardware - a collective term used to describe the physical components that form a computer. The monitor, CPU, disk drives, memory, modem, and other components are all considered hardware. If you can touch it, it is hardware.

HIS (hospital information system) - an integrated computer-based system to store and retrieve patient information including laboratory and radiology reports.

IDE (integrated device electronics) - a type of interface used for hard disk drives that integrates the control electronics for the interface on the drive itself. Its purpose is to increase the speed at which information can be transferred between the hard disk and the rest of the computer.

IMACS - Image Management and Communication System.

Image - a computer's digital representation of a physical object.

Image compression - reduction of the amount of data required to represent an image. This is accomplished by encoding the spatial and contrast information more efficiently, discarding some non-essential information, or both.

Interface - the connection between two computers or parts of computers. It consists mainly of electronic circuitry.

Irreversible compression - some permanent alteration of digital image data. This is sometimes referred to as lossy.

ISDN -integrated services digital network. A switched network with end-to-end digital connection enabling copper wiring to perform functions such as high-speed transmission which frequently require higher capacity fiberoptic cable.

K (kilo) - stands for the number one thousand. It is used primarily when referring to computer storage and memory capacities: for example, 1 kbps = 1024 bytes.

LAN (local area network) - computers in a limited area linked by cables that allow the exchange of data.

Laser film scanner - a device that uses a laser beam to convert an image on x-ray film into digital image data.

Leased line - same as a dedicated line.

Lossless - see reversible compression.

Lossy - see irreversible compression.

M (mega) - stands for the number 1 million. It is used primarily when referring to computer storage and memory capacities; for example, 1 MB = 1 million bytes. 1 MB = 1024 thousand bytes or 1000 kbytes.

Matrix size:
Small - defined as images from CT, MRI, ultrasound, nuclear medicine, and digital fluorography.

Large - defined as images from computed radiography and digitized radiographic films.

Memory - electronic circuitry within a computer that stores information.
Modem - a device that converts digital signals from a computer to pulse tone signals for transmission over telephone lines.

Monochrome monitor - a computer display in which an image is presented as different shades of gray from black to white. (see also gray-scale monitor)

Mouse - an input device that allows the computer user to point to objects on the screen and execute commands.

Operating system - software that allocates and manages the resources available within a computer system. UNIX, MS-DOS, Macintosh, and Windows are examples of operating systems.

Optical disk - a computer data storage disk used primarily for large amounts (GB) of data.

PACS - Picture Archiving and Communication System.

Peripheral - a device that is connected to a computer and performs a function. Scanners, mouse pointers. printers, keyboards, and monitors are examples of peripherals.

Phosphor - the coating on the inside of a CRT or monitor that produces light when it is struck by an electron beam.

Pixel (picture element) - the smallest piece of information that can be displayed on a CRT. It is represented by a numerical code within the computer and displayed on the monitor as a dot of a specific color or intensity. An image is composed of a large array of pixels of differing intensities or colors.

Protocol - a set of guidelines by which two different computer devices communicate with each other.

RAM (random access memory) - a type of temporary memory in a computer in which programs are run, images are processed, and information is stored. The amount of RAM that a computer requires varies widely depending on the specific application. Information stored in RAM is lost when the power is shut off.

Resolution - the ability of an imaging system to differentiate between objects.

Reversible compression - no alteration of original image information upon reconstruction. This is sometimes referred to as lossless.

RIS - Radiology Information System.

Roam and zoom - the ability to select and magnify a region in the display.

ROM (read memory) - a permanent memory which is an integral part of the computer. Programs and information stored in ROM are not lost when the power is removed.

SCSI (small computer systems interface) - SCSI is an interface protocol that is used to link dissimilar computer devices so that they can exchange data. SCSI interfaces are most common in image scanners and mass storage devices. This type of interface is well suited for imaging applications.

Secondary image capture - the capture in digital format of image data that originally existed in another primary format (e.g., a digital image data file on a CT scanner, or a screen-film radiographic film) through the process of video capture or film digitization.

Software - a name given to the programs or sets of programs that are executed on a computer.

Tera (T) - stands for approximately 1 trillion (10^{12}). It is used primarily when referring to archive storage capabilities; for example, 1 TB-one trillion bytes or 1 million MB or 1000 GB.

Throughput - a measure of the amount of data that is actually being communicated, expressed in bits per second. It is related to the baud rate but is usually somewhat less in value due to non-ideal circumstances. Typically, modems with higher baud rates can attain a higher throughput.

Video capture - the process by which images are digitized directly from the video display console of a modality, such as CT, MRI, or ultrasound. The video signal is converted to a digital signal. This process is more efficient and produces better quality images than scanning films that are produced by the same equipment.

Voxel (volume element, derived from pixel) - a voxel is, as the name would imply, a three-dimensional version of a pixel. Voxels are generated by computer-based imaging systems, such as CT and MRI. Using voxels, three-dimensional simulations of objects can be reconstructed by imaging systems.

WAN (wide area network) - a communication system that extends over large distances (covering more than a metropolitan area), often employing multiple communication link technologies such as copper wire, coaxial cable, and fiberoptic links. The cost of these wide area networks is presently dominated by transmission costs.

WORM (Write Once Read Many times) - a peripheral memory device that stores information permanently.

Appendix 3: Glossary

10BaseT: A method of distributing Ethernet data short distances over ordinary telephone lines.

Address: The physical, or conceptional, location of information within the computer, usually used to refer to memory locations. In Internet parlance, the string of information (human or machine readable) that specifies the location of the information of interest and the computer upon which it is located.

Alias: A name or placeholder for a file, application, destination, or grouping of information. A special recipient name for a group of Internet addresses.

Anonymous file transfer protocol (FTP):   Computer site set to allow public retrieval of files using the login "anonymous."

Applet: A small computer program, written in the Java programming language, that is downloaded and run under the auspices of an Internet browser program.

Application: A group of instructions that tell the computer how to accomplish a task. This is usually a relatively complex set of instructions, which handle a variety of related tasks necessary to accomplish an overall type of task, such as word processing, making a graph, or playing music.

Archie: An information retrieval system for anonymous FTP sites.

Archive: A set of one or more files that have been compressed to save space or speed up transmission over the Internet. Many of these files have names that end in *.zip* or *.sit* depending on the compression program used to create the file.

ASCII: American Standard Code for Information Interchange. A computer code for expressing numerals, letters of the alphabet, and other symbols based on eight bits of binary code.

Attachment: One or more files that are sent along with an electronic mail message.

Audio board/sound card: Some computers require the addition of an additional circuit board to play monophonic or stereophonic sounds. With such a card and a compact disk player, the computer may play music, or utilize sounds embedded within software programs. Many computers require a sound card to play music or transmit voice over the Internet.

Back door: A secret way into a computer that bypasses the normal security procedures.

Backbone: The basic communications link of a network.

Bandwidth: A measure of the amount of information that may be transmitted at a given time. Applied to the Internet in general, but may be applied to any method of information transmission. Often used in off-hand comments about the content of information, such as, "It was a waste of bandwidth," to indicate wasteful or frivolous information.

Baud: A measure of the speed of transmission of information. Originally applied to Teletype information, it is roughly equal to one character per second. Introduced in 1931 and named for the French inventor J.M.E. Baudot.

BBS: Bulletin board system. Electronic bulletins board where messages may be read or posted for others to see.

Binary: Based on two alternatives, such as mathematical base 2. In this base, only two digits represent all numbers: 1 and 0. Like the base 10 that we use every day, position relative to the rightmost digit determines the exponential value of each digit. When summed, the final value is reached. In base 10 (B_{10}) the expression 123 is equivalent to 1 times 10^2, plus 2 times 10^1, plus 3 times 10^0. Since $10^2 = 100$, $10^1 = 10$, and $10^0 = 1$ this gives us $100 + 20 + 3 = 123$. In base 2, the same principle applies except that the base number used for each place is 2. Therefore, $1011_2 = 1$ times 2^3, plus 0 times 2^2, plus 1 times 2^1, plus 1 times 2^0 or $8 + 0 + 2 + 1 = 11_{10}$.

Bit: The smallest unit of information. A unit of information that may have two states (e.g., 1 or 0). This may represent any information that may have two mutually exclusive conditions, such as true or false, on or off, light or dark, etc. In a binary string, it represents one digit. In computing, a bit is a single 1 or 0 stored in the computer.

Bookmark: An Internet address (URL) that is stored in a folder for future reference. In Netscape, the file is called the bookmark file, while Internet Explorer calls the file favorites.

Bounce or bounce back: An electronic mail message is returned as undeliverable. This may happen if you have a bad address or if the receiving party cannot receive mail at that time (e.g., server is off line).

Byte: A collection of bits, usually in multiples of two, such as 4, 8, 16, or 32. This represents the width (in bits) of a computer "word." The larger the byte a computer can use, the more information that may be contained in a single word. A byte that is four bits wide can contain only 16 (2^4) possible combinations of 1's and 0's. By contrast, a 32-bit byte can contain over 4 million combinations (2^{32}).

Cable modem: A modulation demodulation device that uses conventional TV cable to transmit data at high speeds.

CD-ROM: A storage device that uses lasers to store and read data. Typical CD-ROM sizes range from 640 to 700 MB or 74 to 80 minutes.

CDR: CD-ROM recordable. A recordable type of CD-ROM. This type of storage disk can be recorded onto once, in which cases the data are permanently recorded.

CDRW: CD-ROM recordable and rewritable. A recordable type of CD-ROM that can be erased and can be recorded onto many times.

Channel or chat room: One of several terms used for an area where Internet users may exchange live text messages. Channels and chat rooms often have themes that provide a common thread or topic of conversation. Some channels or chat rooms have a monitor to keep order; some do not.

Client: A computer that uses the services of another computer (a server).

Clock speed: A timing "clock" coordinates all of the activities of the computer. All activities take place as discrete steps that are kept in cadence by this clock. As a result, the faster the clock speed, the more instructions or activities the computer can accomplish in a give amount of time. Because of the amount of data transferred and manipulated during and Internet session, a computer with a fast clock speed is required.

Cookies: A small file left on your computer (in the hard drive) that saves information about you and your interaction with the distant computer Web site. This information may contain when you last visited, your shirt size, type of computer you use, or your preference in books. The next time you visit that Web site, it can retrieve the cookie and use the information to customize its interaction with you.

CPU: Central processing unit. This is the "thinker" that makes the computer function. This is the chip that interprets the software instructions, performs operation such as addition and subtraction, stores and requests information from memory, and makes logical decisions. It is this branching to various parts of a computer program based on conditions that could not be known at the time the program was written that makes computers so powerful. Like clock speed, the more powerful the CPU, the faster and easier Internet travel becomes.

Cursor: An indicator (flashing box, line, underline, arrow, or other image) displayed on the computer monitor that tells the user where the next action will take place.

Demon: An automatic utility program that runs in the background of a computer. Often used to respond to requests for information or to handle incoming mail.

DICOM: Digital imaging communications in medicine.

Digest: A collection of messages about a specific topic prepared by a mailing list moderator.

Digital camera: A camera that uses a CCD detector and storage devices to capture and store images. Instead of using conventional photographic film, a digital camera will produce electronic images.

Document: A body of data that may be interpreted by an application. This may be information about the look and content of a letter, how to draw a picture or graph on the screen, the contents of a spreadsheet, or any other body of data that an application may need to carry out its task. Generally these data are specific to a set of circumstances that the user has specified and are not required for the normal operation of the application. (See Resource.)

Domain name: Name of a computer system that is registered with the Internet. Can be made up of subdomains such as geographical or organizational subdomains.

Download: To obtain a file of data or a program from a remote computer.

DSL: Asymmetric digital subscriber line. A method of transmitting data at high speeds over telephone lines. In this system, the speeds of transmission in one direction or the other may differ.

DVD: Digital video disk or digital versatile disk. A higher capacity storage device than CD-ROM that also uses specialized lasers to store and read data.

Dynamic rerouting: Ability of a network to direct communications around a damaged connection to still reach the intended recipient.

E-mail: Electronic mail.

Electronic medical record (EMR):   The portion of the patient encounter not captured by conventional information systems, typically ambulatory data including chief complaint, progress notes, medications, allergies, H&P, etc. Commonly referred to as the EMR. Often times this term is used to connote the entire set of electronic medical data on a patient.

Electronic patient record (EPR):   The combination of conventional medical information systems data (lab, radiology, ADT, etc.) and the (ambulatory) electronic medical record.

EPROM: Erasable programmable read-only memory. A type of ROM that may be altered by the user or machine but retains the information when the power is removed. This is useful for storing some types of information, such as start-up preferences, security passwords, etc.

Ethernet: A fast local network originally developed by the Xerox corporation.

Eudora: A mail-handling program for either Windows or Macintosh computers.

FAQ: Frequently asked question.

File: Like a document, this is a collection of data. The term is less specific and may apply to a document, application, or other collection of related data.

Film recorder: Similar to a printer, this device uses instructions passed from the computer to draw information onto film using a very narrow beam of light, passed through one of three primary filters. Just as a printer "draws" a letter on the paper, film printers "draw" information onto film, which may then be developed to reveal the image.

Firewall: A combination of hardware and software used to keep unauthorized users from accessing parts or all of a computer's files or connections.

Flame: To post angry or insulting messages. This may lead to a flame war or (fruitless) exchange.

Forum: A newsgroup.

FreeNet: A computer network that brings together the resources of a community or campus and is available free of charge.

FTP: File transfer protocol. A set of specifications that support Internet file transfer.

Gateway: Computer system that acts as a point of access to allow information to move back and forth between networks. Often used when the networks involved use different protocols.

GIF: Graphics interchange format. A form of graphics file compression developed by CompuServe to be used for file transmission over the Web. These files are generally larger than files using the JPEG format.

Gigabyte: One billion bytes of data.

Gopher: A way of organizing and categorizing certain types of information on the Internet.

Graphics tablet: A type of information input device that uses a pen or other cursor devices on a special surface or tablet to draw, write, or select options. This type of input device is very commonly used for graphic arts and design work.

GUI: Graphic user interface. The "desktop" metaphor used by Macintosh computers and the Windows series of operating systems. These interfaces use icons such as folders and sheets of paper to take the place of directories and data documents to facilitate use by those not familiar with the details of computer structure or function.

Hacker: A person who attempts, for fun or other purposes, to use unauthorized means to enter and use other computers. Generally applied to computer entry via the Internet.

Header: Information placed at the start of an electronic mail message that assists with routing and the display of the message.

HIS: Hospital information system. The computer system used to store all patient data, including laboratory data and other relevant medical data. This usually is on a mainframe computer.

Home page: A Web page about a person or organization. Often used to mean the first screen of information that someone sees when accessing a Web site.

Host: A synonym for any computer connected to the Internet, generally at a remote location.

HTML: Hypertext markup language. A computer language used to transmit information about the display of graphics, text, music, and other information. The language allows commands to be embedded that instruct the computer what information is to be displayed, in what manner, and where that information may be found. The language allows references to information to take the place of the information itself, resulting in smaller files and faster information transfer. Most Web browsers interpret HTML instructions as part of the process of creating the Web page we see.

HTTP/HTTPs: Hypertext transfer protocol. The way the World Wide Web transfers pages over the Internet. The additional "S" indicates an encrypted or secure transmission protocol.

Hyperlink: A special set of instructions transparent to the user that allow a word or line of text to be associated with a Web page or Web site. When users click on that word or phase, they will be taken to that location.

Hypertext: Text that contains embedded links to other data.

Initialization string: A series of characters that are sent as commands to a modem that establish the settings to be used. The exact commands required will be contained in the modem's user manual.

Internet: The name for a group of worldwide computer-based information resources connected together.

InterNIC: Internet Network Information Center. A central repository of information about the Internet and site where domain names may be registered. (http://www.internic.net)

Intranet: A term used to describe an Internet-type network that is within a physical boundary, such as a radiology department. An intranet uses similar or the same protocols as the Internet but does not necessarily have to be connected to the Internet.

I/O device: Input/output device, or a device that allows communications between the user and the computer. This may take many forms: a keyboard, display screen, printer, scanner, modem, film recorder, or mass storage device such as a hard, floppy, or compact disk drive. Some of these communicate in only one direction, while others are capable of two-way communication. Collectively, many of these devices are referred to as peripheral devices. The most common I/O devices involved in using the Internet are modems or network interface cards.

ISDN: Integrated services digital network. A very high-speed connection (usually a dedicated telephone line) used to link computers to the Internet or to connect one computer to another.

ISP: Internet service provider. A third-party provider that supplies access and temporary Internet addresses to users by way of dial-up modem connections. In many cases, the provider also supplies additional services such as e-mail accounts, databases, chat rooms, etc.

IT: Information technology. A colloquial term applied to the field of technology and information infrastructure.

Java: A programming language that allows small applications to be transmitted across the Internet and run independently of the computer platform used. These programs generally perform small tasks related to the display of information in Web browsers.

Joystick: A pointing device based on the two-dimensional motions of a control stick. Common in the early days of computing and in game playing, now relegated mainly to the world of video games.

JPEG: Joint Photographic Expert Group. Compression standard used to format pictorial information. Files formatted using this standard usually have names that end in .jpg or .jpeg. Usually pronounced "JAY-peg."

Jughead: An information retrieval system for a specific Gopher site.

Keystroke logger: A program that automatically keeps a file of everything that is typed from the keyboard.

LAN: Local area network. A term used to describe the geographic span of a computer network. A LAN usually is the size of the radiology department.

Link: A hypertext pointer to another file or Web site that may be invoked by pointing and clicking on the appropriate portion of the displayed Web page. The term also refers to the text-based reference to the URL provided in the Web page instructions themselves.

LINUX: An emerging operating system that is based on an open source code.

Listserv: Listserver, the most common computerized mailing list administration program.

Login ID: Unique identifying character string assigned to a user of a computer system.

Lossy/lossless: Compression methods that reduce the size of images using various methods. Lossy involves loss of data; lossless preserves all of the original data.

Luddite: A person who believes that the progress brought by machines is dangerous to the public good.

Lurk or **lurking:** Listening in on a mailing list or newsgroup discussion without replying.

Lynx: A text-based Web browser program.

Mail server: A computer that provides electronic mail services.

Mailbot: A computer program that automatically sends or answers electronic mail.

Mailing list: A collection of Internet addresses that facilitates an electronic discussion group.

MAN: Metropolitan area network. A term used to describe the geographic span of a computer network. A MAN usually is the size of an entire city.

Mass storage device: One of several types of devices that store large amounts of data in the form of files. Most common are hard disk and floppy disk drives. Compact disk players that can read computer files stored on CD-ROM disks also come under this heading. Internet surfing requires a large amount of storage space for both intermediate files used by the Web browser to display each page and by the audio, video, and picture files often transferred and stored by the user.

Megabyte: One million bytes.

Memory: A nonspecific term for the area in which information is stored. The term may be applied to the working memory of the computer, such as RAM, ROM, etc., or to mass storage devices such as disk drives.

MIDI: Musical Instrument Digital Interface. A protocol for transmitting music as a series of commands (notes) rather than as the sounds themselves, allowing the receiving device to play them in their own way. Many electronic instruments can send or receive MIDI information.

MIME: Multipurpose Internet Mail Extension. A system used to send text, pictures, programs, and other nontext information as a part of electronic mail.

Mirror: One or more computers that share (mirror) the same information so that the load on popular sites may be spread out to improve access speed. In some systems, a mirror site may be selected automatically and the user is unaware of its use; in others, users may choose the mirror site they wish to use.

Modem: Derived from the terms "modulate" and "demodulate," a modem uses telephone or other communications routes to transmit data. The speed and protocol by which this is done varies, but shares the common feature of converting digital information into a varying tone that may be carried by the communications path and interpreted by the receiving modem, which converts the tone back into digital information.

Mosaic: A Windows-based Web browser program that was the predecessor of most of the advanced browsers in use today.

Mouse: A type of pointing device that moves on the physical desktop to move a cursor on the computer screen. The mouse usually has one or more buttons or switches with which to indicate choices.

MPEG: Motion Picture Experts Group. A standard (now entering its fourth iteration) for how video information is compressed and transmitted.

Multimedia: An overused term for anything that uses more than one medium, such as sound, images, movies, and the like. The term is not specific and may be applied to almost any type of software product.

Netscape: A Web browser program available for both Macintosh and PC (IBM compatible) computers.

Network: Two or more computers connected together so that information can move between them.

Newbie: A newcomer to the Internet, just a step up from "clueless newbie."

Newsgroup: A collecting site for messages about a specific theme.

Newsreaders: Programs used to access a newsgroup, such as rn, tn, nn, and tin.

Node: A computer (host or server) on the Internet.

OCR: Optical character reader. A type of scanner and software that allow a printed page to be "read" into the computer and interpreted as a string of characters rather than an image.

Packet: A chunk of information traveling as a bundle over the Internet. The packet contains information about its origin and destination, file type and size, and additional information about confirmation of receipt, etc.

PACS: Picture archiving and communication system. A term used to describe the system that enables filmless radiology. The principal components of a PACS are the archive, the workstations, and the networks that connect them.

Parallel port: A pathway for information transfer in which the data are moved as a byte or word over a series of wires that simultaneously have a sequence of 1's and 0's.

Password: String of characters secretly chosen to verify that you are the valid user connected with a specific user ID.

PCMCIA/PCI: Personal Computer Memory Card International Association/Peripheral Component Interconnect. First developed as a standard for add-on memory for portable and palm-top computers, this now refers to a standard that allows chip-based peripheral components to be plugged directly into a special port to provide special functions such as fax, modems, or memory. These are mainly found on newer portable machines.

Pixel: Picture element. The smallest unit used to make a picture on the monitor screen or printer output. The smaller the pixel, the more detailed the picture; the more pixels, the larger the image.

Plug-in: A small computer program that is added to another (usually your browser program) that adds special functionality or a special type of information, such as music or video.

Pointing device: Any one of several types of devices used to move a cursor on the computer display. Common types are the mouse, track ball, trackpad, joystick, or graphics tablet.

POP: Point of presence. Literally, a connection to the Internet. Generally refers to an Internet service provider (ISP) that provides access to the Internet by temporarily assigning an Internet address from a group owned by the provider.

Port: A pathway in and out of the physical box that contains the computer. This path may transfer raw information, or information that has already been processed into a different form, such as a telephone or video signal.

Portal: A Web site that serves as an entry point to the Internet. A portal is usually thematically based. For example, for a radiologist, a radiology portal would provide all the necessary information needed to access data, cases, and information about radiology.

PPP: Point-to-point protocol. A protocol that allows the use of someone else's Internet presence on a temporary basis. Internet service providers allow a user to connect to the Internet using this protocol.

Printer: Any device that converts computer information and places it on a printed page. This may be accomplished by the use of a sophisticated typewriter-like device (daisy-wheel printer), a group of small pins that draw letters and images as a set of finely spaced dots (dot-matrix printer), sprayed small droplets of ink ("jet" printers), heated elements that transfer wax (thermal transfer), or drawing the image onto a copier-like drum using a small beam of light ("laser" printers). Speed, quality, and the possibility of color printing vary with the technology used.

Protocol: Agreed upon rules for communications between devices (generally computers, modems, or fax machines). These include signals that mean "start," "stop," "got it," "send again," "all done," etc.

Push technology: Methods that allow information posted on a Web site to be sent automatically to others without waiting for them to request it. This is somewhat analogous to broadcasting the information, but unlike broadcasting, the sender is assured the information will be received.

QuickTime: A video file format widely used on the Internet. Originally developed by Apple Computer but available for all platforms.

RAM: Random access memory. This is the memory that may be used by the user and software to store information on a temporary basis. Any location may be addressed at any time. This memory is "volatile" and the information stored there will be lost if the power is lost or if some other information is placed in the same location.

Resource: A set of data, often stored in the same location as the application itself, that is used by the application to accomplish a specific part of its work. Resources may be icons, sounds, images, information, or portions of a dialog directed toward the user. This information is generally only for the use of the application, and may not be addressed or used by the user under normal circumstances.

RIS: Radiology information system. The computer system used to schedule, report, and bill all radiologic studies. This conventionally is on a mainframe computer.

ROM: Read-only memory. This is memory that contains information used by the computer operating system that is independent of the software program that is running. This information is placed there by the computer designers and is permanently place into memory at the time the chips are manufactured. This memory is not lost when the power is turned off, allowing this type of memory to help in the start-up process.

Router: A computer that connects two or more networks

RVU: Relative value unit. A novel term applied to a radiologic study quantifying its value in terms of other radiologic studies.

Scanner: A device used to convert physical materials into computer renderings. This may be in the form of a picture "copied" from a printed source, the image of a printed page, or through the use of special software, a transcript of the printed page that may be manipulated in a word processing program.

SCSI: Small Computer Serial Interface ("skuzzy"). This is a high-speed pathway for communicating between the computer and special input-output devices, most notably memory storage devices such as hard disks, CD-ROM drives, input devices such as scanners, and the like.

Search engine: A program used to find information on the World Wide Web.

Serial port: A pathway for information transfer in which the data is moved as a series of 1's and 0's. This is the most common point of connection for a modem.

Server: A computer system used up to host functions that a client can log into and execute. For example, a "Web" server will host the Web pages of a Web site, and a client will access these with a Web browser.

Shareware: Computer programs that are widely distributed on the honor system. You may try the program at no charge, but it is understood that you will send a use or registration fee if you decide to keep and use the program.

SIMM/DIMM: Single in-line memory module/dual in-line memory module. A small, single- or double-sided circuit card that may be inserted into a computer to provide additional RAM.

SLIP: Serial Line Internet Protocol. A protocol that allows the use of someone else's Internet presence on a temporary basis. Internet service providers allow a user to connect to the Internet using this protocol.

SMTP: Simple Mail Transfer Protocol. The system used to pass mail from one Internet computer to another.

Socket: The logical "port" used by one computer program to connect to another program running on the Internet.

Software: The group of instructions that the computer uses to carry out one or more tasks.

Spam: The act of sending unrequested electronic mail. Generally restricted to mass-mailing types of mail or newsgroup postings.

Surf: To wander around sites on the World Wide Web looking for interesting material.

TCP/IP: Transmission Control Protocol/Internet Protocol.

Telemedicine: The practice of medicine at disparate geographic locations from the immediate location of the physician or patient.

Teleradiology: The transmission and interpretation of images at remote locations.

Telnet: A program used to connect to a remote computer.

Terminal emulation connection: The process that allows your computer screen and keyboard to control a remote computer.

Trackball: A pointing device that moves the computer cursor based on the movements of an upturned ball, somewhat analogous to an overturned mouse.

Trackpad: A pointing device that senses the movement of a finger over its surface.

Upload: To move a file of data or a program to a remote computer.

URL: Uniform Resource Locator, a standardized method for referencing an item on the World Wide Web, including a complete description and its location.

Usenet: User's network, made up of all machines that receive network newsgroups.

User ID: User identification, synonymous with login ID.

Veronica: An information retrieval system for Gopher sites.

Video card: Many computers require a separate card (electronic circuit board) to produce the video signal sent to the monitor. This card often contains its own dedicated memory (VRAM{) to allow more colors, higher resolution. or faster displays.

Virtual memory: A technique that allows space on a hard disk to act as if it were part of the computer's active (RAM) memory.

Virus: Small computer programs that "infect" a computer of files by starting its own operation without the permission or knowledge of the operator. These programs make copies of themselves, allowing them to infect other computers. Viruses vary from those that put a surprise message on the monitor, to those that will erase data or corrupt files. A number of commercial products exist to help identify, remove, or "immunize" against viruses. The use of specialized languages that has made Internet browsers and other tools so powerful (such as Applets and Java Scripts) now opens the possibility of viral transmission across the Internet.

VR: Voice recognition, now an antiquated term that has been replaced by *speech recognition.* This is a technology that converts the spoken word into text on a computer.

VRML: A language used to build virtual reality pages on the World Wide Web.

WAIS: Wide area information servers. A way of categorizing and organizing certain types of information on the Internet.

WAN: Wide area network. A term used to describe the geographic span of a computer network. A WAN usually is the size of an entire hospital.

War dialer: A program that is used to dial a series of telephone numbers. Often used by hackers to look for computer modems.

WAV file: A format for transmitting sound files. File names generally end with .*wav.*

Web browser: An information retrieval program for the World Wide Web that can interpret and display hypertext documents.

Web page: A set of HTML instructions that display information on a Web browser.

Web site: A collection of Web pages that usually are created around a specific common subject.

WebTV: A method of connecting to the Internet using television cables to carry the signal and the user's home television to display the information.

World Wide Web (WWW):   A hypermedia-based system that lets users browse through information stored in different formats.

WYSWYG: "What you see is what you get." Refers to print and other documents that appear on the computer display in the same way that they will when printed to paper or a film recorder.

XML: Extensible Markup Language. A set of extensions to the HTML language that expand functionality.

Zip disk: A trade-named removable disk based on technology introduced by Iomega, which can store approximately 100 megabytes of information. The term, like Kleenex and Xerox, has become generalized to refer to high-capacity small diskettes.

Index